Earn CME while you learn!

Up to 150 *AMA PRA Category 1 Credits*™ available with the MedStudy 13th Edition Internal Medicine Review Core Curriculum

Release Date: November 1, 2008   Expiration Date: November 1, 2011

This CME credit is provided by MedStudy. To apply for CME credit, you must complete the **Verification of Credit** form and Product **Evaluation** found on the following pages. Then submit this completed form and evaluation, along with the $40 CME processing fee, to MedStudy. All necessary contact information is included on the Verification of Credit form.

Please note: CME credit is available **only** to the original purchaser of this product – issuance of CME credit is subject to verification of product ownership.

The Release Date for the MedStudy 13th Edition, Internal Medicine Review Core Curriculum is November 1, 2008. To be eligible for CME credit, you must study the content in the books and submit your Verification of Credit form and Evaluation no later than November 1, 2011.

Accreditation / Designation Statements

MedStudy is accredited by the Accreditation Council for Continuing Medical Education (ACCME) to provide continuing medical education for physicians. MedStudy designates this educational activity for a maximum of 150 *AMA PRA Category 1 Credits*™. Physicians should claim credit only commensurate with the extent of their participation in the activity (one hour = one credit).

Learning Objectives

As a result of participation in this activity, learners should be able to:

- Integrate and demonstrate increased overall knowledge of Internal Medicine

- Identify and remedy areas of weakness (gaps) in knowledge and clinical competencies

- Describe the clinical manifestations and treatments of diseases encountered in Internal Medicine and effectively narrow the differential diagnosis list by utilizing the most appropriate medical studies

- Apply the competence and confidence gained through participation in this activity to both a successful Board exam-taking experience and daily practice

Target Audience / Method of Participation

Internists or other physicians preparing for the ABIM certification or recertification IM exam – or who simply want to refresh their knowledge of Internal Medicine – should thoroughly read each section of the Core Curriculum two to three times for maximum learning and integration. Pay special attention to yellow-highlighted text, which is considered to be the must-know facts for the ABIM Board certification and recertification exams. Use Quick Quiz questions to self-assess your learning (answers to these questions are found in the yellow-highlighted text, or in Figures and Tables), as well as brief review questions at the end of each subspecialty section. Review figures and tables to reinforce your text reading and to see concise summaries of interrelated facts and clinical examples in key topic areas.

Authors / Editors

Robert A. Hannaman, MD
President & CEO
MedStudy Corporation
Colorado Springs, CO

Candace Mitchell, MD
Co-Director, MedStudy ABIM
    Recertification Review Course
Associate Director of Education
MedStudy Corporation
Colorado Springs, CO

J. Thomas Cross, Jr., MD, MPH
Co-Director, MedStudy ABIM Recertification
    Review Course
Director, MedStudy ABIM Intensive
    Certification Review Course
Vice President of Education
MedStudy Corporation
Colorado Springs, CO

Specialty/Subspecialty Reviewers & Advisors

ALLERGY & IMMUNOLOGY

Breck Nichols, MD, MPH
Assistant Professor
Division of Allergy/Immunology
Director, Medicine and Pediatrics
    Residency Program
Los Angeles County and University of
    Southern California School of Medicine
Los Angeles, CA

Larry W. Williams, MD
Associate Professor of Pediatrics
Division of Pediatric Allergy
    and Immunology
Duke University School of Medicine
Durham, NC

CARDIOLOGY

Michael R. McMullan, MD, FACC
Staff Cardiologist
Jackson Heart Clinic
Jackson, MS

David Abrams, MD
Staff Cardiologist
Clinical and Invasive Cardiology
Austin Heart Clinic
Austin, TX

DERMATOLOGY

Margery Atkins Scott, MD
Clinical Professor of Dermatology
Department of Dermatology
Eastern Virginia Medical School
Norfolk, VA

ENDOCRINOLOGY

Robert Richards, MD
Associate Professor of Medicine
Department of Medicine,
    Section of Endocrinology
Louisiana State University
    Health Sciences Center
New Orleans, LA

Fredric B. Kraemer, MD
Professor of Medicine
Chief, Division of Endocrinology,
    Gerontology, and Metabolism
Stanford University School of Medicine
Palo Alto, CA

GASTROENTEROLOGY

Norton Greenberger, MD
Clinical Professor of Medicine
Harvard Medical School
Brigham and Women's Hospital
Boston, MA

GENERAL INTERNAL MEDICINE

(Covers Radiology, Pharmacology,
Statistics, Geriatrics, Ethics,
Ophthalmology, Preventive Medicine, ENT,
Women's Medicine, Psychiatry, Poisoning)

Doug Paauw, MD
Professor of Medicine
Rathmann Family Foundation
Endowed Chair in Patient-Centered
    Clinical Education
Head, Section of GIM,
    Department of Medicine
University of Washington
    School of Medicine
Seattle, WA

HEMATOLOGY / ONCOLOGY

Fred Schiffman, MD
Professor and Vice Chairman of Medicine
The Warren Alpert Medical School
Clinical Director of the Lifespan
    Comprehensive Cancer Center
Brown University
Providence, RI

Anthony Mega, MD
Associate Professor of Clinical Medicine
Co-Director of the Hematology/Oncology
    Fellowship Program
The Warren Alpert Medical School
Brown University
Providence, RI

Angela Plette, MD
Hematology / Oncology Fellow
The Warren Alpert Medical School
Brown University
Providence, RI

INFECTIOUS DISEASE

Alan Morganstein, MD
Glendale, CA

J. Thomas Cross, Jr., MD, MPH
Vice President of Education
MedStudy Corporation
Colorado Springs, CO

NEPHROLOGY

N. Kevin Krane, MD, FACP
Vice Dean for Academic Affairs
Professor of Medicine
Chief, Clinical Nephrology
Department of Internal Medicine
Tulane University School of Medicine
New Orleans, LA

NEUROLOGY

David Lichter, MD, FRACP
Professor of Clinical Neurology
Department of Neurology
School of Medicine and Biomedical Sciences
State University of New York at Buffalo
Buffalo, NY

PULMONARY MEDICINE

Robert A. Balk, MD
Professor of Medicine
Director, Division of Pulmonary
    and Critical Care Medicine
Department of Medicine
Rush University Medical Center
Chicago, IL

RHEUMATOLOGY

Lisabeth Scalzi, MD
Assistant Professor of Medicine
    and Pediatrics
Division of Rheumatology
Milton S. Hershey Medical Center
Pennsylvania State University
Hershey, PA

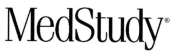

Initial Certification • Recertification • CME

P. O. Box 38148
Colorado Springs, CO 80937
1-800-841-0547

DISCLOSURE SUMMARY

MedStudy adheres to the ACCME's Essential Areas, Elements, Policies, and Criteria, including the Standards for Commercial Support. Disclosures of authors/reviewers and commercial relationships have been documented below, and any perceived conflicts of interest have been resolved by MedStudy's CME Physicians Oversight Council before publication. This pertains to any entity producing, marketing, re-selling, or distributing health care goods or services consumed by, or used on, patients. The resulting certified activity was found to provide educational content that is current, practice-based, and free of commercial bias.

I.   The following reviewers have openly disclosed inclusion of discussion of any off-label, experimental, or investigational use of drugs or devices in their provided content and/or have indicated any affiliation with organizations that may have interests related to such content:

REVIEWER	AFFILIATION/DISCLOSURE(S)
Norton Greenberger, MD	Consultant – Johnson & Johnson
Michael R. McMullan, MD, FACC	Speakers' Bureau – Bristol-Myers Squibb, Sanofi-Aventis
Larry W. Williams, MD	Grant/Research Support – Novartis, Ception Therapeutics
	Speakers' Bureau – AstraZeneca, Sanofi-Aventis
Alan Morganstein, MD	Consultant – Abbott
	Speakers' Bureau – Wyeth, Ortho-McNeil
	Off-label use of nitazoxanide and rifaximin for *C. difficile* diarrhea in refractory cases
Robert Richards, MD	Off-label use of bromocriptine and cabergoline to treat prolactinoma in pregnancy; and metformin to treat PCOs (all considered to be standard of care)
Lisabeth V. Scalzi, MD	Off-label use of rheumatology medications that are considered standard of care

II. The following authors/reviewers have documented they have nothing to disclose:

David Abrams, MD	N. Kevin Krane, MD	Doug Paauw, MD
Robert Balk, MD	David Lichter, MD, FRACP	Angela Plette, MD
J. Thomas Cross, Jr., MD, MPH	Candace Mitchell, MD	Margery Scott, MD
Robert A. Hannaman, MD	Anthony Mega, MD	Fred Schiffman, MD
Fredric Kraemer, MD	Breck Nichols, MD, MPH	

III. The following reviewer(s) have received requests but have not provided disclosure information at this date: None

IV. Good Practices Agreement: The author and all reviewers have also signed a Good Practices Agreement affirming that their content contributions are based upon currently available, scientifically rigorous data; that the content is free from commercial bias; and that clinical practice and patient care recommendations presented in the content are based on the best available evidence for these specialties and subspecialties.

Provider Disclosure

Title of Activity: 13ᵗʰ Edition Internal Medicine Review Core Curriculum

In accordance with ACCME (Accreditation Council for Continuing Medical Education) accreditation Essentials, Elements, Criteria, and Policies, MedStudy Corporation documents the following with regard to MedStudy's 13ᵗʰ Edition Internal Medicine Review Core Curriculum:

MedStudy **does not** have a financial interest, arrangement or affiliation with any commercial organization that may have a direct or indirect interest in the subject matter of this activity. This includes any entity producing, marketing, re-selling, or distributing health care goods or services consumed by, or used on, patients. Furthermore, MedStudy complies with AMA Council on Ethical and Judicial Affairs (CEJA) opinions that address the ethical obligations that underpin physician participation in CME, 8.061, "Gifts to physicians from industry," and 9.011, "Ethical issues in CME."

Autosomal Recessive
Hemochromatosis
Alpha 1 - Antitrypsin Deficiency

Autosomal Recessive
Hemochromatosis
Alpha 1 - Antitrypsin Deficiency

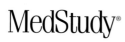

CME Application

IMPORTANT: You must complete both sides of this form and submit it to MedStudy to receive CME credit. **CME credit is available only to the original purchaser of this product.** Issuance of a CME certificate is subject to verification of product ownership.

P.O. Box 38148
Colorado Springs, CO 80937
Phone: 1-800-841-0547, ext. 3
FAX: 1-719-520-5973

Verification of Credit

13th Edition Internal Medicine Review Core Curriculum

Release Date: November 1, 2008   **Expiration Date: November 1, 2011**

MedStudy is accredited by the Accreditation Council for Continuing Medical Education (ACCME) to provide continuing medical education for physicians. MedStudy designates this educational activity for a maximum of 150 *AMA PRA Category 1 Credits™*. Physicians should claim credit only commensurate with the extent of their participation in the activity (one hour = one credit).

My signature on this document certifies my participation in the CME activity:
MedStudy's 13th Edition Internal Medicine Review Core Curriculum.

I have logged _____ hours and claim _____ *AMA PRA Category 1 Credits™*. **(maximum credits: 150)**

Signature:_____ Date: _____

Printed Name: _____

Street Address: _____

City/State/Zip Code:_____

Telephone:_____ Fax: _____

Email*:_____ Specialty: ❑ General IM ❑ IM/Peds ❑ Other _____

Affiliation: ❑ Physician   ❑ Resident Physician   ❑ Non-Physician _____

Exact name of **original purchaser** (individual or institution) ❑ Same as above ❑ Other_____

Please select the method of delivery for your completed CME certificate. (*E-mail preferred.)
❑ Mail   ❑ Fax   ❑ E-mail (Please ensure that your e-mail will accept attachments from MedStudy.)

CME processing fee: $40

Payment method: ❑ Check or money order (payable to MedStudy)
                           ❑ Visa ❑ MasterCard

FAX to: (719) 520-5973 (include credit card information), or

Mail to: MedStudy
              P.O. Box 38148
              Colorado Springs, CO 80937

Card # _____ Expiration Date _____

Authorized Signature on Credit Card Account _____

Now complete the Evaluation on next page (required)

IMPORTANT: ALL questions on this Evaluation MUST be answered before CME credit can be awarded.

CME Learning Activity Evaluation
MedStudy 13th Edition Internal Medicine Review Core Curriculum

Please rate the following regarding your use of the product:

	STRONGLY AGREE	AGREE	NEUTRAL	DISAGREE	STRONGLY DISAGREE
The topics presented met my personal expectations	1	2	3	4	5

This product helped me...

	STRONGLY AGREE	AGREE	NEUTRAL	DISAGREE	STRONGLY DISAGREE
Integrate and demonstrate increased knowledge of Internal Medicine	1	2	3	4	5
Identify and remedy areas of weaknesses or other gaps in knowledge and clinical competencies	1	2	3	4	5
Describe the clinical manifestations and treatment of diseases encountered by the Internist and effectively narrow the differential diagnosis list utilizing the most appropriate medical studies	1	2	3	4	5
Better apply the competence and confidence gained through participation in this activity to both a successful Board exam-taking experience and daily practice	1	2	3	4	5
The topic-by-topic format, Quick Quizzes, and other features made the books a viable mode of instructional delivery	1	2	3	4	5
The content was balanced and free of commercial bias	1	2	3	4	5
The activity offered a reasonable balance of diagnostic and therapeutic options	1	2	3	4	5

Please rate the quality of coverage for the following specialty/subspecialty topic areas:

	EXCELLENT	GOOD	FAIR	POOR	N/A
Allergy & Immunology	1	2	3	4	5
Cardiology	1	2	3	4	5
Dermatology	1	2	3	4	5
Endocrinology	1	2	3	4	5
Gastroenterology	1	2	3	4	5
General Internal Medicine	1	2	3	4	5
Hematology	1	2	3	4	5
Infectious Disease	1	2	3	4	5
Nephrology	1	2	3	4	5
Neurology	1	2	3	4	5
Oncology	1	2	3	4	5
Pulmonary Medicine	1	2	3	4	5
Rheumatology	1	2	3	4	5

Regarding your daily practice, did this Core Curriculum provide information you used to change and/or improve your diagnostic and/or treatment of patients? ❏ Yes ❏ No

If yes, please describe these changes as specifically as possible: _____

_____

General comments about this product, MedStudy, and/or the ABIM Boards: _____

_____

How many years have you been in practice? ❏ Resident ❏ < 1 yr ❏ 1–10 yrs ❏ 10–20 yrs ❏ > 20 yrs ❏ Do not practice

Did you use this activity to (check all that apply):

❏ Prepare for Initial Certification ❏ Prepare for Recertification (MoC) ❏ CME ❏ General Review ❏ Other _____

When did you take (or will you take) the ABIM exam? _____ / _____ (mm/year)

Did you pass the ABIM exam? ❏ Yes ❏ No ❏ Don't know yet ❏ Haven't taken it ❏ Did not use product for exam prep

How did you hear about this product? ❏ Brochure ❏ Colleague ❏ Website ❏ Used other MedStudy products ❏ Other

Thank you for completing this MedStudy EVALUATION. **Please return this evaluation with your CME Application.**

MedStudy®

13th Edition

Internal Medicine Review Core Curriculum

Book 1 of 5

Topics in this volume:

Gastroenterology

Infectious Disease

Authored by Robert A. Hannaman, MD
With Candace Mitchell, MD and J. Thomas Cross, Jr., MD, MPH

NOTICE: Medicine and accepted standards of care are constantly changing. We at MedStudy® do our best to review and include in this publication accurate discussions of the standards of care and methods of diagnosis. However, the author, the advisors, the editors, the publisher, and all other parties involved with the preparation and publication of this work do not guarantee that the information contained herein is in every respect accurate or complete. We recommend that you confirm the material with current sources of medical knowledge whenever considering presentations or treating patients.

MedStudy®

13th Edition

Internal Medicine Review Core Curriculum

Gastroenterology

Authored by Robert A. Hannaman, MD

With J. Thomas Cross, Jr., MD, MPH

Many thanks to *Gastroenterology Advisor:*

Norton J. Greenberger, MD
Clinical Professor of Medicine
Brigham and Women's Hospital
Boston, MA

Gastroenterology

Table of Contents

Gastroenterology

Contraindications to GI endoscopy include a recent MI, combative patient, and intestinal perforation.

Esophagogastroduodenoscopy (EGD) is the procedure of choice for:
- evaluation of painful swallowing (odynophagia);
- determining presence of a peptic ulcer—either instead of UGI or when the UGI is equivocal or negative—and always before peptic ulcer disease (PUD) surgery;
- workup of GERD if initial treatment fails, or if there are alarm signals (see GERD);
- UGI bleed workup;
- workup of GI disease during pregnancy;
- dysphagia (after the barium swallow!);
- prn for evaluation of an ingested foreign body; and
- persistent dyspepsia (a normal EGD is necessary for diagnosis of non-ulcer dyspepsia).

Endoscopic retrograde cholangiopancreatography (ERCP): 60% have an elevated amylase after ERCP, and acute pancreatitis occurs in 5–20%. Treat patients with possible bile duct obstruction with antibiotics before ERCP. Indications for ERCP are unclear, but it is often used:
- to find an otherwise undetectable common duct stone,
- to determine the cause of pancreatic duct obstruction,
- to potentially diagnose chronic pancreatitis,
- to rule out primary sclerosing cholangitis (PSC) (but MRCP is better), and
- to treat choledocholithiasis with cholangitis.

ERCP is contraindicated in acute pancreatitis, except in the following conditions:
- impacted gallstones
- lack of clinical improvement of a non-alcoholic, acute pancreatitis
- ascending cholangitis (bacterial infection causing cholangitis)

MRCP (magnetic resonance cholangiopancreatography) can be used to diagnose chronic pancreatitis and is the test of choice for primary sclerosing cholangitis (PSC).

Table 1-1: Causes and Symptoms of Dysphagia

Disease	Main Problem	Symptoms are...	Symptoms precipitated by...
Schatzki Ring	Anatomic	Intermittent	Solids
Stricture	Anatomic	Progressive	Solids, then liquids
Cancer	Anatomic	Progressive	Solids, then liquids
Achalasia	Neurologic	Longstanding	Solids AND liquids
DES	Neurologic	Intermittent	Solids AND liquids (esp cold)
Systemic Sclerosis	Various	Progressive	Solids AND liquids

Retrograde cholangiography visualizes the bile tract (percutaneous transhepatic cholangiography [PTC], U/S, CT scan, and PIPIDA scans are also used). Retrograde pancreatography is used to visualize the pancreatic duct. Colonoscopy is discussed later.

Endoscopic ultrasonography (EUS) is done via a high-frequency ultrasound probe that is passed through the biopsy channel of the endoscope—allowing for exact placement. It is used especially in evaluating pancreatic diseases. It is also used in biliary duct disease when an ERCP would normally be used but is contraindicated (e.g., gallstone pancreatitis and pregnancy).

DYSPHAGIA

The initial act of normal swallowing (deglutition) is a voluntary action that leads to involuntary upper esophageal sphincter (UES) relaxation and epiglottis closure. The smooth muscle in the esophageal body then generates a peristaltic contraction propelling the food bolus distally. The lower esophageal sphincter (LES) relaxes to allow the bolus to enter the gastric fundus.

When swallowing does not proceed appropriately for any reason, this is termed dysphagia. The history often gives important clues as to the etiology of dysphagia. Distinguish dysphasia from odynophagia, where the patient perceives pain as the food bolus traverses the esophagus. The causes of dysphagia can be categorized into 3 types:
1) Transfer disorders: This is due to neurologic deficit, resulting in difficulty transferring food from the mouth to the esophagus and leads to oropharyngeal muscle dysfunction. Symptoms include coughing, gagging, and nasal regurgitating immediately upon swallowing. Causes include CVA, ALS, etc.
2) Anatomic or structural disorders: This is due to an actual physical obstruction of the esophageal lumen.
3) Motility disorders: Trouble with transporting food from the upper esophagus to the stomach. This can be a failure of effective peristalsis and/or failure of LES relaxation. It has endogenous or exogenous causes.

Diagnosis: Always work up dysphagia. Do not use empiric treatment.

1) The barium swallow is usually the first test performed in the workup of dysphagia, unless the etiology is known from past evaluations. It is definitely done as the first test if symptoms are severe or if there is new onset dysphagia with liquids.

Barium swallow is usually done before endoscopy because:
- There is a risk of perforation when endoscoping a patient with diverticula or high-grade obstruction.
- Information from the barium swallow may preclude the need for endoscopy.

notes

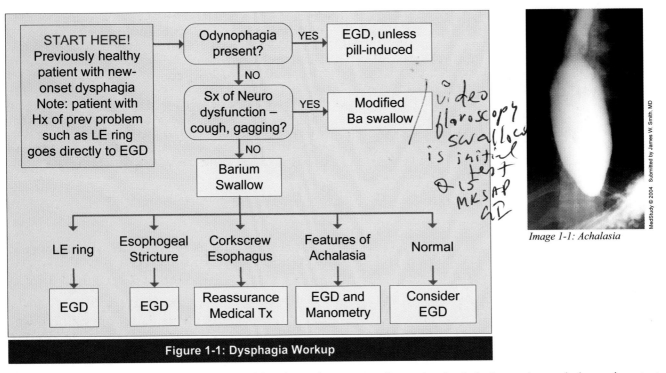

Flowchart:

START HERE!
Previously healthy patient with new-onset dysphagia
Note: patient with Hx of prev problem such as LE ring goes directly to EGD

→ Odynophagia present? → YES → EGD, unless pill-induced

↓ NO

Sx of Neuro dysfunction – cough, gagging? → YES → Modified Ba swallow

↓ NO

Barium Swallow

- LE ring → EGD
- Esophogeal Stricture → EGD
- Corkscrew Esophagus → Reassurance Medical Tx
- Features of Achalasia → EGD and Manometry
- Normal → Consider EGD

(handwritten note: video floroscopy swallow is initial test Θ is MKSAP GI)

Figure 1-1: Dysphagia Workup

Image 1-1: Achalasia

MedStudy © 2004   Submitted by James W. Smith, MD

- Information from the barium swallow provides the endoscopist a general idea of the type and severity of the underlying lesion.
2) EGD generally follows barium swallow if needed, but know that EGD can be done first if the patient has a history of reflux and presents with slight to moderate dysphagia for solids because the pre-test probability is high for stricture secondary to chronic reflux. Esophageal dilation can be done along with the EGD.

3) The third available test is esophageal manometry, which is usually done only if dysphagia persists after negative barium swallow and EGD studies.

Again, workup of dysphagia: 1 = barium swallow, 2 = endoscopy if needed, 3 = manometry studies if needed. See Figure 1-1.

ACHALASIA

Achalasia is of unknown pathogenesis, but it has characteristic and diagnostic features. Neuronal denervation and ganglion cell degeneration of myenteric plexus lead to the following findings:
- No organized peristalsis in the esophageal body.
- The lower esophageal sphincter (LES) has elevated pressure or resting tone.
- The LES does not relax with swallowing.

The characteristic features of the history are:
- dysphagia for solids and liquids,
- long-standing symptoms, usually years,
- regurgitation of food, especially at night, and
- no age or gender predilection.

The diagnosis of achalasia can be made by various tests, usually in this order:
1) Barium swallow: The esophagus will appear dilated and is often fluid-filled. The barium may take a long time to empty into the stomach, even if the patient is upright. There is a "bird-beak" narrowing distally, which represents the tight LES. See Image 1-1.
2) EGD: Generally, the 2nd test ordered; done mainly to confirm the diagnosis and exclude a tumor at the esophagogastric junction.
3) Esophageal manometry: Generally done as a last test to confirm the diagnosis before treatment is offered. This will clearly show the lack of normal peristalsis and the non-relaxing LES.

Remember the 3 tests for achalasia: barium swallow, endoscopy, and manometry.

Also remember pseudoachalasia and secondary achalasia. A tumor at the esophagogastric junction can mimic the history and diagnostic findings of achalasia. Especially consider this diagnosis if onset of symptoms is rapid, patient is > 60 years, and symptoms are progressive and include profound weight loss.

Complications of achalasia include aspiration pneumonia and weight loss.

Focus treatment for achalasia at opening the LES, usually by pneumatic dilation, in which a large, 3–4 cm diameter balloon is inflated within the LES and tears the sphincter open. This balloon is much larger and generates higher pressure than the balloons used to treat esophageal rings and strictures. There is a 5% risk of perforation. Surgical myotomy is

notes

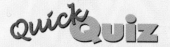

also very effective and can be done via laparoscope. Botulinum toxin is effective in 65% of cases, but requires repeat therapy in 6–12 months. It is an alternative therapy in high-risk patients. Calcium-channel blockers and nitrates have been used in the past with, at best, temporary partial relief.

DIFFUSE ESOPHAGEAL SPASM

Diffuse esophageal spasm (DES) is a simultaneous, non-peristaltic contraction of the esophagus, often precipitated by cold or carbonated liquids. This may be a cause of dysphagia, chest pain, or both. The chest pain is atypical in description—thus, rarely confused with cardiac ischemia. Occult reflux can be responsible for causing esophageal spasm in the absence of typical reflux symptoms.

Barium swallow is usually normal, but may show the classic corkscrew pattern. See Image 1-2.

Manometry confirms the diagnosis by revealing intermittent, simultaneous (non-peristaltic) contractions. LES pressure may be low, normal, or high (i.e., nonspecific).

Endoscopy is rarely helpful. Even in those patients with spasm due to reflux, there is usually no obvious or gross reflux esophagitis. If reflux is considered a possible cause of the diffuse esophageal spasm, order a 24-hour esophageal pH recording or give twice daily proton pump inhibitors (PPIs) for 3 months.

Treatment: Think of this as irritable bowel of the esophagus. Reassurance is the most important part of therapy.

However, if reassurance is not effective or the patient requests specific therapy, recommend these in this order:
1st line: diltiazem or imipramine
2nd line: isosorbide or sildenafil
3rd line: botulinum toxin injection

Obviously, avoiding certain foods, like cold beverages, may be important. PPIs if GERD is suspected (half of pH studies are abnormal). Some patients report benefit from empiric esophageal dilation, although the rationale for this is difficult to understand, and a benefit over placebo is hard to prove.

ANATOMIC OBSTRUCTION

Overview

Anatomic obstruction causes a slowly progressive dysphagia—initially to solids, then to liquids when severe. Depending on the cause, this slowly progressive dysphagia may be intermittent or constant.

In younger patients, it is usually caused by a Schatzki ring (lower esophageal ring), whereas in older patients, it is usually due to cancer (esophageal or extrinsic compression) or stricture.

Lower Esophageal Ring (Schatzki Ring)

The lower esophageal ring (LE ring or Schatzki ring) is a common cause of dysphagia, especially in younger patients. Patients will give a classic history of intermittent solid food dysphagia, especially for meat and bread. They may have to regurgitate the impacted bolus for relief. LE ring is always associated with a hiatal hernia, and reflux may have a role in pathogenesis. However, at endoscopy there is usually no obvious esophagitis. On barium swallow the ring should be 13 mm or less in diameter to cause symptoms. Treatment is dilation using either the bougie method or a through-the-scope hydrostatic balloon. Patients are placed on PPIs after dilation. See Image 1-4.

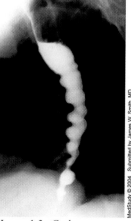

Image 1-2: Corkscrew esophagus

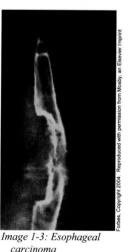

Image 1-3: Esophageal carcinoma

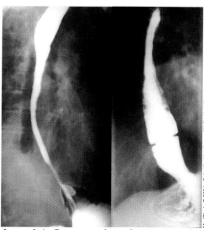

Image 1-4: Severe esophageal stricture on the left, Schatzki ring on the right

notes

Esophageal Stricture

Esophageal stricture presents with a history of constant, not intermittent, dysphagia for solid foods. Usually the stricture is due to a long history of incompletely treated acid reflux. It can also be due to prolonged nasogastric tube placement or lye (rare today, except in those who ingested lye decades ago; these have a chronic stricture and an increased risk of esophageal cancer). Barium swallow shows narrowing usually at the esophagogastric junction. Treatment is dilation. See Image 1-4.

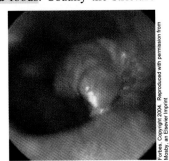

Image 1-5: Esophageal cancer

Forbes. Copyright 2004. Reproduced with permission from Mosby, an Elsevier imprint

Malignant Obstruction

Malignant obstruction can be due to esophageal adenocarcinoma, squamous cell carcinoma, or extrinsic compression from non-esophageal primary cancers. Usually the history is of rapid progression of symptoms: solid food dysphagia to soft food difficulties and finally to problems with liquids. See Image 1-3 and Image 1-5.

Plummer-Vinson Syndrome

Plummer-Vinson syndrome is a rare disorder and results in dysphagia due to a web in the cervical esophagus. It is found in females who have iron deficiency anemia; the reason for this association is unknown. Those with Plummer-Vinson syndrome have a slight increased risk of esophageal cancer.

NEUROLOGIC DYSFUNCTION

Neurologic problems involving the swallowing and/or esophageal peristaltic mechanism cause dysphagia to solids and liquids.

Examples include CVA, Parkinsonism, bulbar palsy (lower motor neuron—ALS, MS) and pseudobulbar palsy (upper motor neuron—ALS).

Bulbar palsy causes dysphagia due to weakness, whereas pseudobulbar palsy causes dysphagia due to disordered contractions. Any type of dysphagia can cause aspiration. This aspiration is often well tolerated and does not need treatment, unless pulmonary problems arise. These patients may complain of choking, gagging, and nasal regurgitation.

If aspiration is suspected, perform a modified or 3-phase barium swallow to confirm the diagnosis. Tracheostomy does not often cure chronic aspiration. A percutaneous endogastric tube (PEG) or endojejunal tube (PEJ) may be required.

Video swallowing studies are also useful in evaluating neurologic dysfunction.

SCLERODERMA

Progressive systemic sclerosis (PSS; scleroderma) is the most common connective tissue disease involving the esophagus. > 80% of patients with PSS have involvement of the esophagus! When the esophagus is involved, the patient has very weak-to-absent esophageal peristalsis. The LES is "wide open" with no tone or pressure, resulting in severe acid reflux damage to the esophagus.

Dysphagia can be due to any one or a combination of the following 3 problems:
1) esophagitis
2) stricture
3) poor motility

So workup requires a barium swallow followed by EGD to look for all three of these possibilities.

If esophagitis is present, begin aggressive PPI therapy. Perform a follow-up endoscopy at 2–3 months to confirm healing and to assure effectiveness of the PPI dose.

Any stricture can be safely dilated using standard techniques.

Note that polymyositis and dermatomyositis can have similar effects on the esophagus.

EOSINOPHILIC (ALLERGIC) ESOPHAGITIS

Primary eosinophilic esophagitis is a chronic inflammatory disorder of the esophagus. It has become increasingly recognized, and its pathogenesis involves interleukin-5 (IL-5) in a central role in concert with eotaxin.

Over 50% of patients have a prior history of respiratory allergies, with a smaller number having food or skin allergies. IgE is elevated in 2/3 of patients.

The leading symptom is recurrent attacks of dysphagia with food impaction. More common in men. On average, patients will have symptoms for 4–5 years before diagnosis. Symptoms are more pronounced in those with a peripheral eosinophilia, which is found in ~ 30% of patients.

The "classic" EGD finding is a scalloped appearance with ridges or rings in the esophagus. Diagnosis is confirmed by esophageal biopsies showing a dense eosinophilic infiltration of the esophageal epithelium (> 20 eos/HPF).

Treatment is difficult. Most recommend referral for allergy testing and avoidance of potential allergens. Fluticasone (bid) or viscous budesonide usually results in a response within a week. Long-term therapy is usually required, and relapses are common when steroids are discontinued. PPI therapy may be helpful in those with concomitant reflux.

MISCELLANEOUS CAUSES OF ESOPHAGITIS

Odynophagia (painful swallowing) is usually due to either pill-induced esophagitis or opportunistic infections.

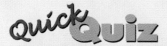

Pill-Induced Esophagitis

Pill-induced esophagitis is most likely when pills are taken with little or no water or before lying down. It is especially seen with doxycycline (teenager with acne), KCl, ASA, NSAIDs, iron, alendronate, and quinidine. The pain can be very severe.

Diagnosis can be made based solely on history! No need for barium swallow or EGD!

Treatment: Stop the offending medicine and reassure the patient that the condition will improve. Educate your patients to take plenty of water with their medications.

Opportunistic Infections

Opportunistic infections can occur in any immunocompromised patient, such as those with diabetes or HIV, but can also occur in an immunocompetent patient on corticosteroids. Commonly it is due to *Candida*, herpes simplex virus, or cytomegalovirus. If you see thrush in the mouth, you can assume that the esophagitis is also due to *Candida*, and treat the patient empirically with fluconazole. If no improvement, or unsure of the diagnosis, then EGD with biopsy is the procedure of choice. Rarely is dilation needed or helpful.

GE REFLUX DISEASE (GERD)

Overview

GE reflux is usually a result of inappropriate, transient relaxation of the lower esophageal sphincter (LES). The transient relaxation is, in part, a reflex caused by recently ingested fat in the duodenum or overdistension of the stomach. Hiatal hernia is another factor—but it is not necessary for reflux.

LES pressure is increased by motilin, acetylcholine, and possibly gastrin. Therefore, drugs that increase these mediators tend to decrease reflux. LES pressure is decreased by progesterone (pregnancy increases GE reflux), chocolate, smoking, and some medications, especially those with anticholinergic properties.

Suspect GE reflux disease (GERD) in patients with a persistent, nonproductive cough, especially with hoarseness, continual clearing of the throat, and a feeling of fullness in the throat. This cough is usually worse at night when the patient is supine.

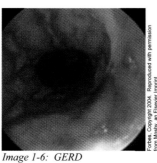

Image 1-6: GERD

Forbes, Copyright 2004 Reproduced with permission from Mosby, an Elsevier Imprint

Most non-cardiac chest pains (70%) are caused by GERD! Most other GI-related chest pains are due to motility disorders. (Note: These pains are not necessarily associated with pyrosis [heartburn] or dysphagia.)

Extraesophageal manifestations of GERD:
- nocturnal cough
- frequent sore throat
- hoarseness, laryngitis, clearing of the throat
- loss of dental enamel
- exacerbation of asthma
- VCD (vocal cord dysfunction)

GERD is associated with two respiratory disorders: asthma and VCD.

Some asthma patients, even without symptoms of GERD, have improvement of their asthma symptoms with GERD treatment. When working up GERD, always ask about asthma symptoms—especially those occurring at night.

Don't assume it is nighttime asthma the patient is complaining of! VCD is a spasming of the vocal cords with associated inspiratory stridor. Patients will tell you they are wheezing at night and may not really know if it is inspiratory or expiratory. VCD is not always due to GERD but is more typically seen in young adults in competitive sports and thought to be more of a stress reaction. About 10% of exercise-induced "asthma" is now thought to be misdiagnosed VCD.

Increased BMI is associated with increased incidence of both GERD and asthma.

Complications: esophageal ulcers, stricture, bleeding, and Barrett esophagus (discussed below).

Diagnosis of GERD

If the patient has only the classic symptom of heartburn, the diagnostic workup starts with a therapeutic trial—EGD is indicated only if this trial fails. (See Figure 1-2).

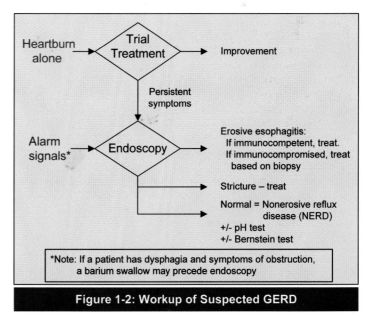

Figure 1-2: Workup of Suspected GERD

notes

Alarm signals in GERD indicating the need for EGD:
- nausea/emesis
- blood in the stool
- family history of PUD
- weight loss
- anorexia
- anemia
- abnormal physical exam
- long duration of frequent symptoms, especially in Caucasian males > 45 years old
- failure to respond to full doses of a PPI
- dysphagia/odynophagia

EGD is also done if Barrett esophagus is suspected.

If the patient has obstructive symptoms, you can do a barium esophagram before endoscopy.

Note: 62% of patients with GERD symptoms have a normal esophagus. This is termed nonerosive reflux disease or NERD!

Conduct the 24-hour esophageal pH monitor for atypical cases, such as:
- refractory symptoms and a normal EGD;
- hoarseness, coughing, or atypical chest pain, but no classic symptoms of GERD; and
- failure to respond to PPIs.

The pH monitor is similar to a Holter monitor in that the patient keeps a diary of symptoms. You then analyze the diary logs and pH monitor results for correlation.

A Bernstein test is now rarely used for diagnosing atypical chest pain; a positive test result is reproduction of symptoms when 0.1 molar HCl is infused into the distal esophageal lumen.

Treatment of GERD

Treatment of mild-to-moderate GERD:

Initial: Raise head of bed*, encourage weight loss of > 10 lb if overweight or recent weight gain*, small meals, no fatty meals in the evening, eat dinner at least 3 hours before bedtime, no sweets at bedtime, stop smoking, and antacids prn (*only these 2 have been shown in clinical trials to be effective; the rest are more "common sense" but not proven by studies to do anything more than placebo). Avoid acidic beverages (e.g., colas, orange juice, wine) and excessive alcohol.

If unsuccessful, try antisecretory drugs: Proton pump inhibitors (PPIs), such as omeprazole, are more commonly used today in clinical practice than H_2 receptor blockers. Although long-term effects of PPIs are unknown, they have been found safe over a 15-year period. PPIs are best if given before breakfast after a nocturnal fast.

Overall healing of patients with endoscopic evidence of esophagitis (not necessarily GERD!):
- placebo: 25%
- H_2 blockers and prokinetic drugs: 50%
- PPIs: 80–95%.

H_2 blockers may heal mild cases of GERD, but treatment of severe GERD (i.e., grade 2 or worse esophagitis) requires PPIs, such as omeprazole, continued indefinitely, unless the patient has corrective surgery.

PPIs in particular are indicated for long-term therapy in patients with EGD evidence of esophagitis.

In patients with GERD symptoms who do not respond to PPIs, check for other medications that may delay gastric emptying and thus promote reflux—especially calcium-channel blockers, antihistamines, tricyclics, and anticholinergics.

Be aware of H^+ rebound if PPIs are stopped abruptly after several months—especially in *H. pylori*-negative patients. Also know: PPI treatment leads to parietal cell hyperplasia, but no dysplasia or neoplasia has been seen.

Consider antireflux surgery (fundoplication, now by laparoscope) in patients with severe GERD because it has a reasonable success rate. Indications are: patients refractory to medical treatment, young patients with severe disease, and as an alternative to long-term PPI. Antireflux surgery is most successful in patients responding to PPIs. However, even after reflux surgery, 60% will still require PPI therapy. With Nissen fundoplication, the lower esophagus is wrapped in a sleeve of the stomach. Side effects of this surgery are bloating, dysphagia, and an inability to belch. You must do a motility study prior to antireflux surgery—because the results may influence the performance of the fundoplication. Patients with very poor peristalsis are at risk for post-operative dysphagia.

Treat peptic strictures secondary to GERD with dilation and then PPIs. Note: Metoclopramide (due to too many side effects) and sucralfate (not very effective) have little use in treatment of GE reflux.

Maintenance therapy consists of PPIs, such as omeprazole, for moderate-to-severe cases. Long-term use of H_2 receptor blockers is usually ineffective.

Be aware that patients with GERD-related cough/hoarseness require much longer treatment and usually higher doses (e.g., bid) for symptomatic improvement of the cough or hoarseness than those with run-of-the-mill heartburn.

BARRETT ESOPHAGUS

Barrett esophagus is a change in cell type—from esophageal squamous to specialized intestinal metaplasia—caused by chronic GE reflux. 10–20% of men endoscoped for chronic reflux have it! And about 2% of women. However, screening for Barrett's is controversial because of the lack of randomized clinical trials that have shown impact on mortality with screening. Saying that, the 2008 guidelines support surveillance screening based on retrospective studies. Also, there are a large number of patients with Barrett esophagus who lack reflux symptoms. According to these guidelines the highest yield for Barrett's is in older (age > 50) Caucasian males with longstanding heartburn.

notes

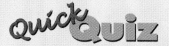
Barrett esophagus is associated only with adenocarcinoma (not squamous). Incidence of adenocarcinoma in patients with Barrett esophagus is 30x the normal rate. Probability of adenocarcinoma is related to the length of Barrett esophagus, presence of a hiatal hernia, degree of dysplasia, and concurrent smoking. Risk of adenocarcinoma is 0.4% per year in patients with Barrett esophagus. Neither antireflux medication nor surgery reverses the epithelial changes of Barrett esophagus or eliminates the cancer risk.

Know the following: The 2008 guidelines are very vague about who should be endoscoped. In general it is based on age, duration of symptoms, and willingness of the patient to adhere to the recommendations. 2 EGDs should be done with biopsy within 1 year. If these 2 EGDs and biopsies are negative for dysplasia, then biopsies should be repeated in 3 years. The finding of low-grade dysplasia on the 1st endoscopy warrants follow-up biopsy within 6 months. If no higher-grade dysplasia is seen on the repeat biopsy, then yearly biopsy is warranted until no dysplasias are present on 2 consecutive annual EGDs with biopsy. If high-grade dysplasia is found on a biopsy, then subsequent biopsy should be done within 3 months. At any biopsy, if high-grade dysplasia is seen with mucosal irregularity, then proceed with endoscopic resection. If high-grade dysplasia is present without mucosal irregularity, some recommend resection while others recommend q 3 month EGD with biopsies.

New imaging modalities (narrow band imaging, optical coherence tomography, etc.) are promising in detecting neoplasia but are not currently recommended by the 2008 guidelines. Additionally, multiple biomarkers have been proposed (genes such as P16, P53, etc.), but are not ready for routine clinical use.

ESOPHAGEAL CANCER

Two types of esophageal cancer: Adeno (slightly > 50%) and Squamous (slightly < 50%).

Adenocarcinoma of the esophagus has been on the rise (from Barrett esophagus) and now occurs more commonly than squamous cell; it occurs in the distal 1/3 of the esophagus. See more in previous discussion.

Squamous cell esophageal cancer usually occurs in the proximal 2/3 of the esophagus, and it is caused by smoking and alcohol (especially hard liquor). It is associated with other cancers of head or neck, and rarely associated with achalasia, lye stricture, or Plummer-Vinson syndrome (see earlier). Smoking and alcohol have a synergistic carcinogenic effect on the esophagus. Incidence of squamous cancer has a marked geographic variation, and its occurrence appears strongly associated with diet and environment.

Diagnosis of esophageal cancer is accomplished with a number of tests. Dysphagia is the usual presenting symptom, so a barium swallow during the workup may suggest cancer. EGD is always done to allow confirmation via biopsy. Use CT scan and endoscopic ultrasound to stage the tumor.

If small and localized, do surgical resection. If large or metastasized, treat with combination chemotherapy (cisplatin + 5-FU) plus radiation prior to surgery. This combination results in a 2-year survival of 38% vs. 10% with radiation alone.

ZENKER DIVERTICULUM

Zenker diverticulum is an outpouching of the upper esophagus. Patients have foul-smelling breath and may regurgitate food eaten several days earlier. This is the most common cause of transfer dysphagia (trouble initiating swallowing) for solid foods, but it can also cause transport dysphagia. These patients are often elderly. Treatment is surgery.

[Note: Know the indications for EGD, ERCP, pH monitor, and motility studies!]

STOMACH

NORMAL PHYSIOLOGY

First, a quick review of normal stomach physiology as it relates to gastritis and PUD. See Figure 1-3. The light green highlight shows the main pathway used in production of gastric acid.

G cells are in the pyloric antrum. Increase in pH and amino acids (from food breakdown) cause the G cells to release gastrin which, like acetylcholine (ACh) and histamine, interacts with specific receptors on the parietal cells in the fundus—stimulating them to secrete (via the proton pump) HCL (gastric acid) into the lumen. Gastrin additionally (and more importantly) stimulates enterochromaffin-like (ECL) cells to produce histamine.

The proton pump is the final common pathway for the action of these 3 receptors, and this is why the PPIs, such as omeprazole, are the strongest anti-gastric-acid drugs.

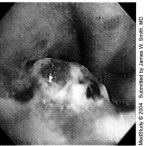

Image 1-7: Barrett esophagus

notes

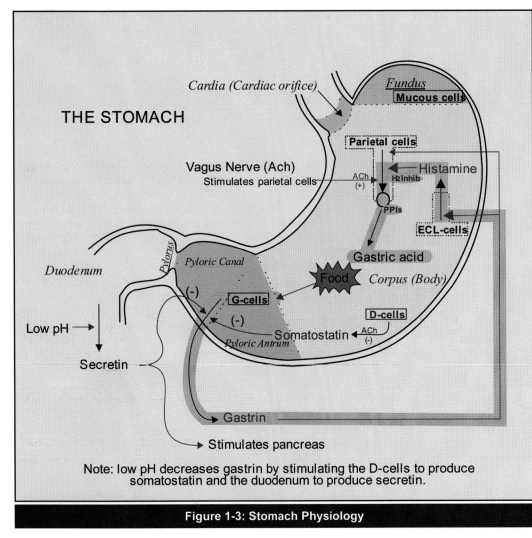

THE STOMACH

Cardia (Cardiac orifice)

Fundus
Mucous cells

Parietal cells

Vagus Nerve (Ach)
Stimulates parietal cells

ACh (+)
H2Inhib
Histamine

PPIs

ECL-cells

Gastric acid

Pyloric Canal

Duodenum

Pylorus

Food
Corpus (Body)

(-)
G-cells
(-)
D-cells

Low pH →

Somatostatin ← ACh (-)

Pyloric Antrum

Secretin

Gastrin

Stimulates pancreas

Note: low pH decreases gastrin by stimulating the D-cells to produce somatostatin and the duodenum to produce secretin.

Figure 1-3: Stomach Physiology

Gastrin is released into the circulation and is therefore an endocrine stimulus for gastric acid release. Gastrin is the dominant mediator of postprandial gastric acid production.

Histamine, released by the ECL cells in the corpus—especially due to gastrin stimulation—has a local paracrine effect via the H_2 receptors of the parietal cells.

ACh (acetylcholine), from the vagus nerve, has a direct neurocrine effect on the parietal cells.

Remember: Parietal cells are affected by endocrine, neurocrine, and paracrine stimuli.

Somatostatin and secretin both decrease the production of gastrin (and therefore gastric acid), and the production of both of these is stimulated by low pH—hence, they are the negative feedback portions of the regulatory mechanism for maintaining stomach pH. A stomach pH < 3 causes production of somatostatin by corpus D cells. Secretin is produced in the duodenum in response to the acidified output of the stomach; it both decreases the gastrin production and stimulates output of bicarbonate from the pancreas. Again, 2 inhibitors of gastrin (and therefore gastric acid) production are somatostatin (low stomach pH) and secretin (low duodenum pH).

Note: In patients with achlorhydria (as in autoimmune gastritis, see below) or pernicious anemia, the serum gastrin level skyrockets because of the loss of this inhibitory effect. If PPIs result in achlorhydria, they can result in a markedly elevated gastrin level (> 500 pg/mL).

Both gastric acid and pepsin (made from pepsinogen in the presence of acid) not only digest food but also attack the mucosal defenses.

Things to know about the mechanical actions of mixing and grinding:
• This is best studied with a gastric emptying scan.
• Only particles < 1 mm can pass the pylorus.
• Peristalsis is activated by a pacemaker.

DYSPEPSIA

Overview

Dyspepsia refers to recurrent upper abdominal pain or discomfort. It can include epigastric fullness, belching, bloating, gnawing pain, and heartburn. It generally does not apply to severe pain. Most are functional or caused by medications (e.g., Fe, ASA, NSAIDs), but if onset is recent and the patient is > 40 years, it is organic until proven otherwise (i.e., do an EGD). For young patients, you can test for *H. pylori* and treat if positive (more below).

Organic causes of dyspepsia include PUD, gastritis, GERD, biliary colic, gastroparesis, pancreatitis, and cancer. EGD is usually normal. Dyspepsia is generally classified by symptoms: GERD-like, ulcer-like (improves on anti-ulcer therapy), and dysmotility-type (improves on promotility drugs, such as metoclopramide). There can also be overlaps in the types.

"Non-ulcer dyspepsia" is defined by recurrent upper abdominal pain with a normal EGD.

So, how do we handle dyspepsia? The following is the overview:
• Work up   • Test and treat *H. pylori*
• Discontinue NSAIDs   • Trial treatment with PPIs
• EGD if there are alarm symptoms or failure of therapy

notes

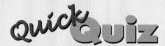
Now we will review more on gastritis and on *H. pylori* infection.

GASTRITIS

Classification Schemes

Gastritis is generally classified by histology or etiology:

1) Classification by histology:
A neutrophil infiltrate is seen in acute gastritis while a lymphocyte and plasma cell infiltrate occur with chronic gastritis. Histologic classification reflects the findings throughout the possible life of the disease:

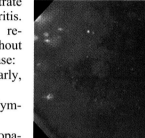

Image 1-8: Acute gastritis

- superficial gastritis (early, neutrophils)
- atrophic gastritis (mid, lymphocytes)
- gastric atrophy (late, gastropathy)—also called metaplastic atrophic gastritis.

Some lump mid and late disease into a single term, "chronic gastritis," which is not quite correct because the inflammation has burned out in the late phase so it is not really a gastritis.

2) Classification by etiology:
Type A: Autoimmune, Atrophic, pernicious Anemia, Achlorhydria. It affects the proximal stomach—fundus and body only. (Note: "Antrum" is not one of the "A" words!) Autoantibodies against both intrinsic factor and the parietal cells cause a progression to pernicious anemia and to achlorhydria, with secondary hypergastrinemia (levels often > 1000 pg/mL). Metaplasia is a universal feature of atrophic gastritis, and it appears before, and is associated with, both pernicious anemia and gastric cancer. Even so, the incidence of gastric cancer is so low with atrophic gastritis that, if there is no cancer or dysplasia on initial endoscopic exam, periodic endoscopic exams are not warranted!

Type B is the most common form of chronic gastritis (80%). It is a curable infectious disease caused by *Helicobacter pylori*. Symptoms and findings can mimic Type A gastritis.
Successful treatment of the infection results in resolution of gastritis symptoms in less than half the patients!
Gastric acid secretion decreases with the increased degree of *H. pylori* gastritis. Oral meds such as ketoconazole and thyroxine require gastric acid for optimal absorption. Fluconazole does not require gastric acid and is usually used as a substitute for ketoconazole in this case. Note: 50% of AIDS patients have decreased stomach acid and are especially prone to ketoconazole failure.
Especially remember thyroxine because this widely used drug was only recently (April 2006, NEJM) shown to require gastric acidity for optimal absorption.

Erosive Gastropathy

Erosive gastropathy, frequently with subepithelial hemorrhage, may be caused by NSAIDs, alcohol, or severe physiologic stress.
Note that gastritis, by definition, means there is an inflammatory response, whereas there is not one in this setting. So, calling this a gastritis, as is commonly done, is technically wrong.

Onset in the ICU suggests stress-related mucosal damage (SRMD), which is due to severe physiologic stress, such as that induced by major surgery or burns. Having severe CNS injuries, being on a ventilator, or having a coagulopathy are also major risk factors. Just about anything works to prevent SRMD: H_2 receptor antagonists, antacids, PPIs, sucralfate, and even early feedings decrease the incidence of erosive gastritis.
Continuous infusion of an H_2 receptor antagonist is the most effective treatment for SRMD. Although it was thought that decreased acidity in the stomach allowed colonization and increased the risk of aspiration pneumonia, it has been shown that there is no increase in aspiration pneumonia with the use of H_2 blockers.

MORE ON H. PYLORI

Overview

H. pylori is linked not only to gastritis but also to PUD, gastric adenocarcinoma, and gastric B-cell (MALT) lymphoma.
Chronic gastritis occurs in all people infected with *H. pylori*, although only a minority have symptoms, and you treat only these symptomatic ones.
Virtually all people in third-world countries are infected with *H. pylori*. In the U.S., the incidence is ~ 50% in older patients and 30% overall. It is usually acquired in childhood. Incidence is decreasing in the U.S.

Testing for H. pylori

Test for *H. pylori* when (know!):
- there is any prior history of PUD, complicated or uncomplicated,
- current findings on EGD show ulcer disease, erosive gastritis, or duodenitis,
- MALT lymphoma, is present, or
- there is a family history of gastric cancer.

The strategy is "test and treat" in dyspeptic patients with age < 55 and no alarm symptoms/features.

notes

H. pylori testing: There are invasive (biopsy specimen) and noninvasive tests. Generally, only patients already targeted for EGD get the invasive tests. Otherwise, noninvasive tests are more cost-effective while still accurate.

Invasive tests:

* The gold standard for *H. pylori* testing is histologic examination of biopsied antral mucosa—which is done only infrequently.
* Urease tests are based on the finding that *H. pylori* breaks down urea into ammonia and CO_2. Urease tests are good for checking for active disease and for response to therapy. These tests are sensitive (95%) and specific (95%). For the CLOtest® and other rapid urease tests (RUT) the biopsy sample is placed on an agar medium containing urea and a pH reagent. Any ammonia then produced causes an increase in pH, which changes the color of the medium. Urease tests are less sensitive if the patient is on a drug that may blunt the effect of *H. pylori* infection, such as PPIs and antibiotics—in such patients, it is appropriate to obtain biopsies for histology with or without RUT or plan testing with a urea breath test or fecal antigen test at a later date after withholding the offending agents for 2-4 weeks.

Noninvasive tests include urea breath testing, fecal antigen tests, and serologic tests:

* Urea breath tests (UBT), which use labeled urea, are the first choice for checking effectiveness of treatment.
* Fecal antigen tests (FAT) are a good method for primary diagnosis and, if the patient is on PPIs, it is the best test for checking for effectiveness of treatment (S&S = 94% & 98%).
* Serologic tests (ELISA—IgG) are inexpensive office tests, but in the U.S. the PPV (positive predictive value) is very poor, which means that a positive test is no better than 50% in predicting the presence of active infection and also poor for checking effectiveness of treatment. As such, serologic antibody tests should be avoided altogether or positive results should be confirmed with a test such as a UBT or FAT. Because of this, serologic testing in the U.S. is discouraged.

Again, PPIs interfere with any urease test (CLOtest and urease breath test) but not with antibody or antigen tests.

Again, PPIs and *H. pylori* gastritis cause decreased gastric acid production, which, in turn, interferes with absorption of some medications (thyroxine, ketoconazole).

H. pylori Treatment

H. pylori treatment is the same whether the patient has gastritis or PUD.

* Treat for 10–14 days. 1 week is insufficient.
* Usually, triple-drug therapy is used—2 antibiotics and a PPI. A good one with an eradication rate of ~ 80% is O-CLAM (omeprazole 20 mg + clarithromycin 500 mg + amoxicillin 1g—all bid x 10 d). Recurrence rate is very low.

Know that the more drugs the better! Single- and dual-drug therapies are ineffective.

Note: *H. pylori* develop resistance to metronidazole and clarithromycin when used alone—so any recent use of these antibiotics precludes their use. Also, regimens that include metronidazole are less effective in the U.S. than Europe—probably because there is increased resistance to metronidazole in the U.S. If 1st course of therapy (PPI and 2 antibiotics) fails to eradicate *H. pylori,* then some recommend PPI + amoxicillin + levofloxacin.

Universal posttreatment testing is not recommended. The accepted indications include the following:

* history of *H. pylori*-associated ulcer
* persistent dyspeptic symptoms despite the test-and-treat strategy
* *H. pylori*-associated MALT lymphoma
* resection of early gastric carcinoma

When confirmation is necessary, testing should be performed no sooner than 4 weeks after the completion of therapy. In general, noninvasive tests should be done for posttreatment testing unless there is a need for repeat EGD.

PEPTIC ULCER DISEASE (PUD)
OVERVIEW

Peptic ulcer disease (PUD) has 4 well-confirmed causes:

1) *Helicobacter pylori* infection is still the most common cause of PUD—especially duodenal ulcer disease (50%, but incidence is decreasing in the U.S.) Lifetime ulcer risk for a person with *H. pylori* infection is 10–15% (higher for men than women). If *H. pylori* can be eradicated, ulcers virtually never recur, and the *H. pylori* recurrence rate is very small. The trouble is getting rid of it! If the ulcer does recur, suspect NSAIDs. See earlier discussion of *H. pylori* testing.

2) NSAIDs cause the majority of peptic ulcers not caused by *H. pylori*. The prevalence of ulcers in patients on NSAIDs is 10–40% (!) although many are < 5 mm and do not cause symptoms. NSAIDs cause both gastric and duodenal ulcers—usually gastric.

If NSAIDs are required, and the patient is having or has had trouble, use:

* enteric-coated NSAIDs
* nonacetylated NSAID (e.g., salsalate = Disalcid®, Salflex®)
* NSAIDs that are non-acidic pro-drugs (e.g., nabumetone = Relafen®)
* NSAID with a PPI or prostaglandin E analog (e.g., misoprostol = Cytotec®). PPIs are superior to H_2 blockers and sucralfate in the prevention of NSAID-induced ulcers.
* COX-2 NSAID (see below)

Risk factors for conventional NSAID-induced PUD include: First 3 months of use, high doses, elderly patient, history of ulcer disease, cardiac disease, concurrent steroids, serious illness, and concurrent ASA (such as for cardioprotection).

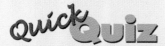

3) High acid-secreting states, such as Zollinger-Ellison (1–3% of duodenal ulcers).

4) Crohn disease of the duodenum/stomach.

What about tobacco? In both gastric and duodenal ulcer disease, smoking exacerbates the ulcer. For non-*H. pylori* ulcers, smoking also decreases the healing rate and increases recurrence and perforation rate. Commonly, these recurrences are asymptomatic.

Previously, the incidence of PUD was higher in men than women, but now the male-to-female ratio is approaching 1. Type of diet, personality, and occupation are not significant etiologic factors! Weight loss is uncommon in PUD. Notes: Alcohol is not ulcerogenic! Corticosteroids alone are not ulcerogenic, but they double the risk of serious NSAID-associated gastrointestinal complication—risk of bleeding may be 10-fold!

DIAGNOSIS OF PUD

The following are currently approved strategies for diagnosing PUD:
• For the younger, healthy patient with classic symptoms, empiric treatment with an H_2 blocker or PPI is acceptable.
• For this same younger, healthy group, *H. pylori* "test-and-treat" is also acceptable.
• EGD is done for all other patients, particularly if melena, heme + stools, or in an older patient.

EGD is always indicated in PUD if these appear in the question:
• associated dysphagia and odynophagia
• follow-up healing gastric ulcer
• UGI bleeding
• foreign body
• abnormal UGI or CT scan

UGI is less sensitive than the EGD and rarely done today to diagnose PUD. If an ulcer is found, serum gastrin levels may be indicated (specifics discussed under the type of ulcer). Diagnose the presence of *H. pylori*, as described in the gastritis section above.

Perforated gastric and duodenal ulcers often cause free air in the peritoneal space, which can be seen on an upright abdominal x-ray. If a perforated ulcer is suspected, do the upright x-ray first! EGD and UGI are contraindicated. Also know that absence of an ulcer crater means there is no risk of hemorrhage, perforation, or scarring!

Know: The pain of an ulcer tends to be gnawing, whereas that of a perforated ulcer is usually severe.

TREATMENT OF NONBLEEDING PUD

Treatment of PUD targets combinations of 3 main strategies:
1) *H. pylori* treatment
2) decrease acid secretion (H_2 receptor antagonists, PPIs)
3) stop exacerbating processes (smoking, taking NSAIDs)

Less frequently used are mucosal protection (sucralfate) and acid neutralization with antacids.

Treat any *H. pylori* infection associated with PUD. This is discussed on pg 1-10.

If the patient tests negative for *H. pylori* infection, and exacerbating factors such as NSAIDs have been addressed, use antisecretory drugs and antacids. Sucralfate is effective in the treatment of non-*H. pylori* PUD, but its qid dosage is a hassle and PPIs are better. Sucralfate binds to the ulcer site, where it binds bile salts and forms a barrier to prevent acid penetration. Sucralfate is often the drug of choice in renal patients because it also binds PO_4.

Stop smoking—it increases risk of recurrence and perforation in ulcers not associated with *H. pylori* or untreated *H. pylori* ulcers.

Indications for surgery in PUD:
• UGI bleed—most common—active bleed unable to stop via endoscopic therapy. Surgery is required in 5% of UGI bleeds—but there are a lot of bleeds.
• Gastric outlet obstruction—initial treatment is balloon dilation. Surgery required in ~ 25%.
• Perforation—laparoscopic repair may be possible.
• Recurrent/refractory ulcers (rare).
• Zollinger-Ellison syndrome (ZES).

notes

DUODENAL VS. GASTRIC ULCER

Duodenal ulcers: Again, the common causes are NSAIDs and *H. pylori*, and only 1–3% are due to increased acid secretion (ZES).

Gastric ulcers not associated with *H. pylori* are treated for 3 months because these heal more slowly than duodenal ulcers. PPIs and misoprostol (a synthetic prostaglandin) are superior to H_2 blockers and sucralfate in the prevention of NSAID-induced ulcers.

Although gastric ulcers were previously thought to increase gastric cancer risk, studies have not shown this to be true! On the other hand, examine all nonhealing gastric ulcers via endoscopy with a cytologic exam of at least 6 biopsy samples to rule out gastric cancer.

BLEEDING PEPTIC ULCERS

NSAIDs

NSAIDs are the leading cause of bleeding ulcers in the U.S. Ulcer symptoms may not occur before bleeding. The bleeding risk is dose-related. As mentioned previously, corticosteroids are not ulcerogenic alone, but they may increase the NSAID-associated bleeding 10-fold!

Risk of bleeding with conventional NSAIDs:
- general population: 1%
- in those using aspirin concurrently as preventive medicine: 1.5%
- history of PUD/UGI bleed: 3%

And NSAID risk is higher if the patient is older than 60 years or a female.

Add cardiac disease to any from this list, and the risk jumps from 3% to 9%.

There is no totally safe dose of aspirin.

Risk of bleeding with COX-2 NSAIDs:
Note the following!
- COX-2 use alone has close to normal risk of GI bleeding (0.5%).
- Baby aspirin use alone has near-normal risk of GI bleeding.
- But COX-2 with low-dose (81 mg) aspirin has same risk as regular doses of NSAIDs (1%)!

COX-2 NSAIDs block the action of cyclooxygenase (COX), an enzyme that converts arachidonic acid to prostaglandin. COX-1 is the constitutive enzyme, while COX-2 is inducible. COX-1 produces protective prostaglandins in the stomach, whereas the inducible COX-2 is involved in inflammatory response. COX-2 inhibitors (celecoxib—Celebrex®, meloxicam—Mobic®) appear to have decreased GI side effects (compared to conventional nonselective NSAIDs), while retaining the antiinflammatory and pain relief effects.

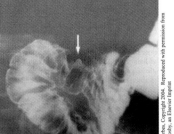
Image 1-9: Small duodenal ulcer on double contrast barium meal

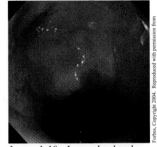
Image 1-10: Large duodenal ulcer

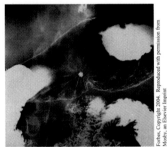
Image 1-11: Benign gastric ulcer on double contrast barium meal

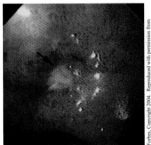
Image 1-12: Similar gastric ulcer seen on endoscopy

Note: All the COX-2 inhibitors appear to have some cardiovascular risk (thrombosis and MIs)—that may vary from one to the other.

COX-2 inhibitors have an FDA-mandated black-box warning label highlighting the potential for increased risk of cardiovascular events and GI bleeding.

Workup of Bleeding Peptic Ulcers

Signs indicating a severe bleed:
- hemodynamic instability
- recurrent red-colored hematemesis or hematochezia
- lack of clearing of gastric lavage effluent

These people also have a high risk of rebleed.

EGD is the diagnostic and treatment procedure of choice for UGI bleed. It should be done emergently if the patient has any of the above findings. EGD is done for two reasons:
1) Treat the current bleed.
2) Assess the risk for rebleed.

EGD findings that indicate increased chance of rebleed:
- larger size of the ulcer
- visible vessels on a non-bleeding ulcer increase the risk for rebleed to 50%
- visible clot = 30%

An ulcer with a clean base (i.e., no bleeding, no clot, and no visible vessels) has a very low chance of rebleed. These pa-

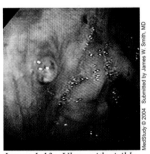
Image 1-13: Ulcer with visible vessel seen on endoscopy

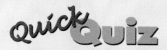
tients are usually sent home the same or next day—unless they have one of the 3 signs of severe bleed mentioned above.

Treatment of Bleeding Peptic Ulcers

What does not work: Gastric lavage does not stop bleeding or prevent rebleeding. IV vasoconstrictors also are ineffective.

The purpose for gastric lavage is to look for blood in the effluent and, if blood is found, clearing of the effluent indicates bleeding has stopped. Remember that blood in the effluent indicates the stomach is the source of bleeding, but no blood does not rule out the stomach!

Increasing the gastric pH to > 6.0 reduces the risk of rebleeding, and PPIs given either IV or orally bid achieve this. Most patients with a bleeding ulcer get prompt IV PPI treatment before endoscopic banding or sclerotherapy, and this is continued until they are able to switch to oral bid therapy.

Initial treatment of actively bleeding ulcers (or adherent clot/visible vessel) show best results with combination therapy consisting of injection (epinephrine, saline, alcohol) followed by either thermal/laser coagulation or a hemoclip.

NON-ULCER CAUSES OF UGI BLEEDS

Osler-Weber-Rendu (hereditary hemorrhagic telangiectasia) causes telangiectasias on the skin, buccal and nasal mucosa, and throughout the GI tract, lungs, and brain. Occasionally AVMs (arterio-venous malformations) occur, and these can rupture and bleed. In the GI tract, these AVMs are usually in the stomach or duodenum.

Peutz-Jeghers syndrome (PJS) causes dark melanin spots on the lips, buccal mucosa, and the hands and feet. Most patients have hamartomatous polyps that can occur anywhere from the stomach to the rectum. These polyps may cause acute or chronic GI bleeds.

ZOLLINGER-ELLISON

Zollinger-Ellison syndrome (ZES) occurs when a gastrinoma, which produces gastrin continuously, causes refractory (usually duodenal bulb and stomach) ulcers and diarrhea +/- steatorrhea. The most common presentation of ZES is diarrhea.

The diarrhea/steatorrhea is from a large volume of gastric juice causing acidification of duodenal contents.

Gastrinomas most frequently occur in the duodenum (~ 50%) or pancreas (~ 25%), and less frequently in the stomach, lymph nodes, and spleen. 90% are found in what is called the "ZE triangle"—which includes the porta hepatis, mid-duodenum, and the head of the pancreas. 80% are of the sporadic form; 20% are associated with MEN type 1.

When to consider ZES? In patients with:
- severe esophagitis and chronic diarrhea,
- ulcer (especially duodenal ulcer) and chronic diarrhea,
- duodenal ulcer and big folds in the stomach (from *parietal* cell hyperplasia),
- recurrent ulcers and no other risk factors,
- recurrent complicated ulcers, and
- post-bulbar duodenal ulcers.

To evaluate ZES, first order a serum gastrin while patient is off PPI therapy. If the gastrin level is elevated in a patient with gastric acid, present workup usually requires abdominal CT, endoscopic ultrasound, and somatostatin receptor imaging.

Treatment: All patients with newly diagnosed ZES without evidence of metastatic disease warrant surgical exploration. 1/3 will be cured by resection of the primary tumor. Even with metastatic disease, treat ZES aggressively with resection of the primary tumor because the mass effect of the tumor tissue can eventually cause problems. A PPI is now the drug of choice for medical treatment of ZES, although the dose is higher than usual.

Remember: Other conditions associated with an elevated gastrin level are vitiligo, renal failure, hyperthyroidism, and achlorhydria caused by PPI use or chronic Type A gastritis (see pg 1-9). Also remember that high gastrin can cause gastric carcinoids. Speaking of which …

GASTRIC CARCINOID

Gastric carcinoids are rare (0.5% of gastric tumors) and usually seen with a chronic hypergastrinemic state, as in:
- autoimmune gastritis/pernicious anemia (type 1), and
- ZES, when it occurs as part of multiple endocrine neoplasia—MEN-I (type 2).

Least often, it is spontaneous (type 3). It may also be associated with vitiligo!

Gastrin is trophic to the enterochromaffin-like (ECL) cells of the stomach, leading to hyperplasia and occasionally to gastric carcinoids. Note: The PPI omeprazole has not been shown to cause carcinoids in humans (10 years worth of data), although it does increase gastrin level.

It is unusual for gastric carcinoids to metastasize or be symptomatic. They are slow-growing and almost never cause carcinoid syndrome. Also see pg 1-22 for more on carcinoids.

GASTRIC CANCER

There are 4 significant malignancies of the stomach:
1) carcinoids (just discussed)
2) adenocarcinoma (most common—95%!)
3) lymphoma
4) GIST (gastrointestinal stromal tumors, e.g., leiomyosarcoma)

There are 2 distinct forms of gastric adenocarcinoma: a proximal diffuse type and a distal intestinal type. The incidence of distal gastric cancer had been decreasing until about 20 years ago; since then, its incidence has been holding steady. The proximal type has been steadily increasing.

The risk factors and associations with gastric cancer include:
• chronic *H. pylori* infection,
• metaplastic (chronic) atrophic gastritis,
• Ménétriér disease (= large stomach folds from epithelial cell hyperplasia), and
• adenomatous gastric polyps (rare).

It appears that distal gastric cancer is most strongly associated with environmental factors, especially:
• a diet low in fruits and vegetables and high in dried, smoked, and salted foods, and
• foods rich in nitrates (animal studies).

Acanthosis nigricans, a reactive skin condition with velvety dark plaques in the intertriginous areas (def: where opposing skin surfaces touch and rub). It is usually due to obesity, but it is also associated with various GI and lung malignancies and conditions that cause insulin resistance. Of the malignancies, acanthosis nigricans is most often associated with gastric cancer.

Note with *H. pylori* infection—some patients may develop MALT (extranodal marginal zone B-cell lymphoma of mucosa-associated lymphoid tissue … er, like I said, MALT). This is diagnosed by EGD with biopsy. When the *H. pylori* infection is treated, the MALT may resolve. Close endoscopic follow-up is necessary.

Neither alcohol consumption nor gastric ulcers has been proven to cause gastric cancer—as previously thought—even though gastric cancer presents as an ulcer.

Diagnosis of gastric cancer: Often an ulcer is picked up on barium contrast study (double contrast is better). If it appears benign, it can be treated. Endoscopy and biopsy are necessary only if it does not heal.

For a non-healing ulcer, endoscopy with multiple biopsies is the diagnostic procedure of choice. Tumor markers, such as carcinoembryonic antigen (CEA) and alpha fetoprotein (AFP), are of no use as early markers for gastric cancer.

Prognosis is determined by stage (TNM classification), using CT scan and endoscopic ultrasound. Because it is largely asymptomatic until advanced, < 10% are found in the early

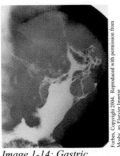

Image 1-14: Gastric cancer—barium meal

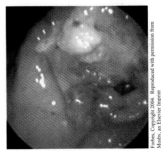

Image 1-15: Gastric cancer

gastric cancer stage (EGC, confined to the mucosa and submucosa, T1N0M0).

5-year survival rate is 85–90% for treated EGC and only 3% for treated invasive, metastatic gastric cancer.

Treatment consists of surgical removal of the cancer and adjacent lymph nodes. Adjuvant combination chemotherapy prolongs survival. Adjuvant radiotherapy is investigational.

OTHER GASTRIC SYNDROMES
POSTGASTRECTOMY SYNDROMES

Overview

Postgastrectomy syndromes include dumping syndrome, blind loop syndrome, and afferent loop syndrome.

Dumping Syndrome

Dumping syndrome consists of postprandial vasomotor symptoms: palpitations, sweating, and lightheadedness. There are 2 types. The early type occurs 30 minutes after eating and is of uncertain etiology. The late type occurs 90 minutes or more after eating and is probably due to hypoglycemia. Both types are treated identically: restriction of sweets and lactose-containing foods, and frequent small meals.

Blind Loop Syndrome

Blind loop syndrome is bacterial overgrowth in a loop manifested by fat and B_{12} malabsorption, and a low D-xylose absorption test (low bacterial overgrowth and with small bowel mucosal problems).

Afferent Loop Syndrome

With a gastrojejunostomy, an anastomosis is formed between the stomach and the jejunum. The "afferent loop" is the portion that was bypassed and through which bile and pancreatic fluids still flow toward the jejunum. Occasionally these patients get "afferent loop syndrome." They present with abdominal bloating and pain 20 minutes to 1 hour after eating; vomiting often relieves symptoms. The emesis is often bile-colored. Many believe the cause is an incompletely draining afferent loop, which fills with the biliary and pancreatic secretions.

notes

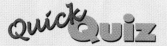
Gastroparesis in Diabetics

Highly variable gastric emptying is seen in diabetics. Emptying may be slow, normal, or fast. However, long-term diabetics tend to develop slow gastric emptying (gastroparesis). This occurs much more commonly in Type 1 than in Type 2.

Blood glucose > 200 mg/dL has been shown to result in decreased antral motility and delayed gastric emptying. Hyperglycemia may also have a negative long-term direct effect on gastric motility.

Conversely, slowed gastric emptying itself tends to increase blood glucose because of the delay of insulinemic and glycemic responses to the carbohydrates.

So we have a vicious spiral and the way to minimize the spiral is to keep tight control of glucose levels.

More on Gastroparesis

Gastroparesis (gastric stasis) is a motor dysfunction with nausea, vomiting, and early satiety, as well as a predisposition for bezoars. It is usually caused by:

• autonomic dysfunction—diabetic neuropathy, amyloid neuropathy; and

• an infiltrative process of the smooth muscles—scleroderma, amyloidosis.

Other causes are all nerve related: CNS disorders (stress, MS, Parkinsonism, tumor), spinal cord injuries or spinal cord ganglion problems, and post-vagotomy. Hyperglycemia slows gastric emptying short-term and possibly long-term and is a factor in diabetic gastroparesis (in addition to the autonomic neuropathy).

Workup of suspected delayed gastric emptying requires you rule out obstruction first. Then diagnosis is confirmed with a radioisotope-labeled solid meal.

Treat with good hydration and nutrition, tight control of blood glucose, and metoclopramide. Erythromycin stimulates gastric motility (it is very similar in structure to motilin) but is less useful as a long-term therapy.

INFLAMMATORY BOWEL DISEASE
COMMON FACTORS

Inflammatory Bowel Disease (IBD) comprises Crohn disease (CD) and ulcerative colitis (UC). In both types, family members are at increased risk of IBD, and the patient has an increased risk of GI cancer—but the risk of cancer is much higher in long-standing UC than in CD.

Toxic megacolon is a complication in both, so a barium enema is contraindicated in both types if the patient is having an acute exacerbation of UC or CD.

Infectious colitis, early CD, and UC can appear identically on sigmoidoscopy. Stool examination for WBCs, O&P, C&S, and *C. difficile* toxin assay are part of the initial workup. Refer to Table 1-2 as you review CD and UC.

Smoking is associated with both CD and UC, but not in the way you might think. Smokers are more likely than the normal population to develop CD, while UC is infrequent in smokers (only 10% of UC patients are smokers)!

Colonoscopy is the usual method used to asses IBD. Barium enema is not used anymore.

The main drugs used to treat IBD include:
• sulfasalazine,
• mesalamine (5-aminosalicylate or 5-ASA preparations),
• olsalazine,
• prednisone,
• budesonide (Crohn disease only),
• metronidazole,
• azathioprine and its metabolite, 6-mercaptopurine, and
• infliximab, adalimumab (monoclonal antibody to TNF-α).

Methotrexate and cyclosporine are also available.

TREATMENT OVERVIEW FOR IBD

Sulfasalazine is split, by bacterial action in the colon, into sulfapyridine and mesalamine (5-amino salicylic acid). Mesalamine is the active component of sulfasalazine—hence, sulfasalazine is ineffective for CD of the small bowel. The other breakdown product, sulfapyridine, is absorbed in the colon, acetylated in the liver, and excreted in the urine. Sulfapyridine is a highly reactive sulfa moiety, which is responsible for most of the side effects of sulfasalazine, such as reversible infertility in men, leukopenia, and headache.

Mesalamine (5-aminosalicylic acid, 5-ASA) is normally rapidly absorbed from the upper digestive tract, but different oral formulations release mesalamine into the distal ileum and colon. For colon disease, it is given either rectally—as an enema (proctosigmoiditis) or suppository (for proctitis only)—or in a formulation designed to delay absorption of the drug. One interesting formulation is olsalazine, which is an aminosalicylic acid dimer that requires colonic azo-reduction (as does sulfasalazine) to reduce into 2 molecules of aminosalicylate in the colon.

notes

Metronidazole is beneficial for perianal abscesses and fistulas in CD. Combined with a 5-ASA analog, it is useful as maintenance therapy for CD. Long-term use is hampered by the side effect of peripheral sensory neuropathy.

Budesonide is an enteric-coated corticosteroid that releases mostly in the ileum and ascending colon. It metabolizes in the liver to inactive products. It has a 90% first-pass effect—thus, much fewer systemic side effects than prednisone. It is used specifically for small bowel CD. As with other corticosteroids, bone mineral density should be monitored yearly. At this point, it is uncertain whether budesonide has less effect on bone density than prednisone.

6-mercaptopurine and azathioprine (which metabolizes to 6-MP) are prednisone-sparing drugs useful in both Crohn and UC, but they usually take 3–4 months to show an effect. Also, because these 2 drugs have bone marrow suppressive effects, monitor CBC monthly. There is no report of increased malignancy with long-term use of either drug.

Infliximab (Remicade®) and the newer adalimumab (Humira®) are chimeric and humanized (respectively) monoclonal antibodies to TNF-α. They are given for moderate-severe Crohn disease, fistulous Crohn disease, and refractory UC. Know that TB may reactivate with usage…but the most common side effect is URIs.

Note: Monoclonal antibodies (mAb) are identical antibodies derived from clones of a single parent cell. The standard recombinant DNA procedure produces mouse (murine) Ab. The human body reacts against these foreign Ab with an inflammatory response. To overcome this, a portion of mouse DNA that codes for the binding site is combined with human DNA. The result is a chimeric (human-murine) Ab or a humanized (mostly human) Ab. The more human, the less reaction. Monoclonal Ab's generic names always end in "mab" (mAb, get it?).

Drugs proven to decrease the relapse rate in CD are azathioprine, 6-mercaptopurine, MTX, and also infliximab (but only for infliximab-induced remission), while all the standard drugs decrease the relapse rate in UC! Mesalamine drugs and corticosteroids are good for inducing remission in CD but not maintaining it.

Stopping smoking decreases relapse rate in CD and increases it in UC.

Use in pregnancy:
FDA risk category B: Metronidazole, prednisone, and sulfasalazine (and probably its derivatives 5-ASA and olsalazine—but these have not been given an FDA risk category yet).

CROHN DISEASE

Overview

Although most patients present with Crohn disease (regional enteritis) in their 20s or 30s, the disease can present at any age. There is even a second, smaller peak of incidence in 70–80-year-olds. The incidence of CD is increasing. There is an increased risk of GI cancer with CD, especially with long-standing disease (> 20 years); screen long-term CD patients every other year for cancer.

CD is more indolent than UC. Because of this, it is less responsive to treatment, and it is harder to get these patients off steroids. Patients with CD are more likely to have perianal fistulae and abscesses. They are also more likely to have strictures, inflammatory masses, and associated obstruction. One big problem with CD is the high rate of recurrence. It was once thought to be 50% at 10 years, but this is the symptomatic recurrence rate. Radiologic/endoscopic recurrence rate is 75% at 3 years!

Osteoporosis is common in Crohn disease. About 70% have abnormal bone density—due to chronic disease and/or steroids.

Diagnosis

CD is diagnosed by finding patchy, focal, and aphthous ulcers and deep transmural ulcers (called "Crohn craters"), with occasional strictures and fistula formation. Granulomas, infrequently found on biopsy specimen of these ulcers, are pathognomonic.

A tetrad to remember for "Crohn colitis:" rectal sparing, skip lesions, perirectal disease, and contiguous ileocolic disease. These patients may get fever, abdominal pain, and systemic symptoms. One classic but uncommon feature of CD is the "string sign," which may be seen in the terminal ileum during a small bowel follow-through. The terminal ileum is so edematous and/or fibrotic that the lumen is compressed and shows up as a "string" of contrast. The edema pushes the rest of the bowel away so the "string" shows up well. If you see

Table 1-2: Comparison of CD and UC		
	Crohn Disease	**Ulcerative Colitis**
Lesions	Focal, skip, deep	Shallow, continuous
Clinical course	Indolent	More acute
Prednisone*	Less responsive	Very responsive
Granulomas	Pathognomonic	None
Rectal Involvement	Rectal sparing in 50%	Rectum ALWAYS involved
Perianal Disease	Abscesses, fistulas	None
Small Bowel Involvement	> 50%	Backwash ileitis in < 10%

For flares. Not for long-term maintenance therapy.

notes

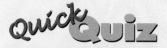
this narrowing of the lumen elsewhere in the colon, it is called an apple-core lesion, which suggests cancer. Bowel involvement in CD: 30% colon only, 40% small bowel only, and 30% both.

Initially, a definitive diagnosis cannot be established in up to 15% of patients with IBD. Serologic tests (p-ANCA and ASCA, anti-saccharomyces antibody) can be useful in indeterminant cases. p-ANCA is associated with UC and ASCA with CD.

Extraintestinal Manifestations in CD

The extraintestinal manifestations occur only in CD involving the colon. These manifestations are identical to those of UC, which involves only the colon. So, these are discussed under UC on pg 1-18.

Terminal Ileum Problems in CD

Problems related to disease/resection of the terminal ileum are found in CD—but not in UC. These problems include
- calcium oxalate kidney stones (if steatorrhea present),
- gallstones,
- B$_{12}$ deficiency,
- hypocalcemia (from vitamin D malabsorption),
- bile acid-induced diarrhea, and
- nutrient malabsorption.

What type of gallstones occur? Probably not what you think. Previously it was thought that cholesterol gallstones formed in this situation because of the loss of bile salts and the resulting bile became supersaturated with cholesterol, but now it appears that this is probably not the case. Pigment gall-stones are the usual type, and the risk appears to correlate with the amount of ileal disease or resection.

Bile acid-induced diarrhea is usually the cause of diarrhea in Crohn patients when < 100 cm of distal ileum is resected. Some of the bile acids escape absorption in the terminal ileum and go on to stimulate colonic salt and H$_2$O secretion by the colon. Treat with bile acid sequestrants (e.g., cholestyramine), which bind and inactivate the bile acids.

When > 100 cm of distal ileum is resected, the patient gets steatorrhea from greatly decreased proximal gut concentration of bile salts (synthesis does not keep up with GI loss with the loss of distal ileum resorption). Treat these patients with a low-fat diet. Sometimes the low-fat diet does not allow them to get enough calories. In this case, give them supplemental medium-chain triglycerides (MCT).

Treatment Overview for CD

See more detail on these medications on pg 1-15.

Medical treatment of CD: sulfasalazine, 5-amino salicylate (5-ASA, mesalamine—slow-release formulations), olsalazine, corticosteroids, metronidazole, azathioprine (and its metabolite, 6-mercaptopurine), and infliximab (Remicade®). See Table 1-3. [Know!]:

- In general, treatment for mild disease is a slow-release oral 5-ASA formulation with progression to other drugs if response is not adequate. 5-ASA analogues are more effective in CD with colon disease only vs. ileal or ileocolic disease.
- Prednisone is more effective in UC than CD—again, probably due to the indolent nature of CD. In CD, prednisone is more effective than sulfasalazine when CD affects only the small intestine. Prednisone is best used only for flares; long-term use (> 3 months) should be discouraged because of side effect issues.
- Budesonide is a second-line drug for mild-to-moderate CD localized to the ileum.
- Infliximab (Remicade®) is a chimeric IgG monoclonal antibody (mAb) to tumor necrosis factor-α (TNF-α), which is helpful in patients refractory to corticosteroids, and especially in patients with fistulas without high-grade obstruction. It also facilitates withdrawal from corticosteroids. Before starting this agent (or adalimumab, below), screen all patients for tuberculosis by checking a PPD. The most common adverse reactions are development of a positive ANA in 55% and URIs in 32%. There is a heightened risk of tuberculosis while on therapy. Additionally, lymphoma and multiple sclerosis have been described in recent reports.
- Adalimumab (Humira®) has the same mechanism of action and indications as infliximab. It has a lower risk of anti-drug antibody formation than infliximab because it is a humanized mAb rather than chimeric.

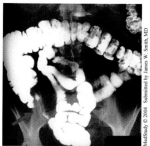

Image 1-16: Crohn colitis with "string sign" in RLQ

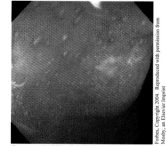

Image 1-17: Crohn proctitis with patchy aphthous ulcers

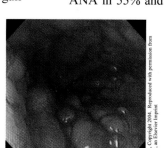

Image 1-18: Crohn colitis

notes

- Metronidazole is effective, especially for fistulas and perianal CD (used for UC only when there is fulminant disease with peritonitis). Combined with a 5-ASA analog, it is useful as maintenance therapy for CD. Again, long-term use is hampered by neuropathy.
- Ciprofloxacin is also occasionally used for fistulous or perianal Crohn disease.
- 6-mercaptopurine (6-MP) and azathioprine are used with Crohn patients who cannot be weaned off prednisone. Note: Long-term treatment with 6-MP and azathioprine has been shown to decrease recurrence rates in CD.

Like 6-MP and azathioprine, mesalamine and olsalazine also probably decrease the relapse rate in CD. Prednisone and metronidazole do not affect relapse rate.

Surgery & Recurrence in CD

Surgery is only for intractable disease and specific serious complications. Previously, 60% of Crohn patients required surgery in the first 5 years and then again after ~ 8 years. These numbers are decreasing with medical therapy (esp. 6-MP, infliximab). The incidence of recurrence after surgery depends on:
- site—ileocolic is highest, and
- nature of the complication—obstruction, perforation, and abscess have higher incidence and rates of recurrence.

Essentially, the worse the disease is where you cut, the more likely is the recurrence at that site. Colectomy and ileostomy provide the best results for Crohn colitis when there is no ileal inflammation (> 60% have no recurrence).

Treatment Scenarios for CD

Colon only: sulfasalazine, mesalamine enemas, or olsalazine. Sulfasalazine is about $25/mo vs. $200–$300/mo for mesalamine and other drugs. Therefore, sulfasalazine is the first choice—then 5-ASA drugs, if required, because of intolerance to the side effects of sulfasalazine.

Any ileum or small bowel involvement: slow-release mesalamine.

Only ileum or small bowel involvement: slow-release mesalamine or budesonide.

Fistula or perianal: infliximab by IV infusion, metronidazole, or ciprofloxacin. 6-MP also used.

Steroid-dependent: 6-MP, azathioprine, mAb.

Corticosteroids are a first-line drug for incomplete acute small bowel obstruction. Otherwise they are used for flares and only if there is inadequate response to the 5-ASA drugs.

Note: Be sure to screen CD patients for osteoporosis. About 70% have abnormal bone density due to chronic disease and/or steroids.

ULCERATIVE COLITIS

Overview

Ulcerative colitis (UC) consists of uniform, continuous mucosal inflammation with shallow ulcers extending proximally from the rectum. There is usually a sharp margin between the area of involvement and the normal mucosa. The area of involvement tends to remain the same from the time of diagnosis, but does extend more proximally in 10%.

65–75% of UC patients are p-ANCA–positive, although this test is of little use clinically (low sensitivity & specificity). ESR and C-reactive protein (CRP) are often elevated.

The main symptoms of UC are abdominal pain and bloody diarrhea. Clinical course and degree of involvement are variable—from mild ulcerative proctitis (rectal area only) with minimal symptoms to severe colitis of the entire colon with bad cramps, liquid stools containing blood and pus, anemia, extraintestinal manifestations (below), and constitutional symptoms. Tenesmus (painful anal sphincter spasm with no bowel movement) and constipation may be the major symptoms with ulcerative proctitis.

You must rule out the infectious causes of colitis: *E. coli* O157:H7 (EHEC), *Shigella, Salmonella, Yersinia, Campylobacter, C. difficile*, and amebiasis. Especially *Campylobacter*—since it can have a chronic, relapsing course that mimics UC.

Consider *C. difficile* infection in a flare-up—it is usually thought of as an acute disease, but it can manifest as diarrhea 1–3 months after antibiotic use!

Diagnosis is made with colonoscopy or sigmoidoscopy.

Extraintestinal Manifestations

Extraintestinal manifestations of IBD are usually seen in IBD patients with colitis (so they are usually associated with UC, although they can be seen in CD involving the colon).

"JSEM" is the mnemonic for diseases seen with colonic disease (colitis): **J**oint, **S**kin, **E**yes, **M**outh. These extraintestinal manifestations of UC include:
- skin lesions—E. nodosum and pyoderma gangrenosum—which correlate with disease activity,
- RF-negative peripheral polyarthritis,
- iritis/episcleritis/uveitis (HLA-B27+),
- venous thrombosis,
- ankylosing spondylitis (also HLA-B27+),
- pericholangitis, and
- primary sclerosing cholangitis (PSC, HLA-B8+, see pg 1-40).

The complications associated with HLA antigens tend not to improve with improvement of colitis, whereas the other problems mentioned here usually get better as colitis improves!

So, what disease do you think of if a patient with UC develops jaundice, itching, and cholestatic LFTs?

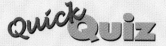

1) Review and know the treatment of CD and UC.

2) Which more commonly involves the rectum—CD or UC?

3) What serological marker may be found in 65–75% of patients with UC?

4) Name the skin lesions associated with UC.

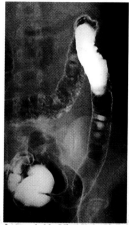

Image 1-19: Ulcerative colitis. Note the loss of haustral pattern and deep penetrating ulcers

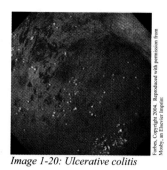

Image 1-20: Ulcerative colitis

The JSEM mnemonic leaves out primary sclerosing cholangitis, the answer to this question! PSC in UC occurs rarely but is a favorite Board question. As with any newly increased LFTs, do an ultrasound first, then do a MRCP to confirm the diagnosis of PSC.

Check LFTs, especially alkaline phosphatase, initially and periodically. If the value becomes 2 x nl and persists, conduct a workup for sclerosing cholangitis.

Cancer in UC

Risk of cancer in patients with UC is high—0.5%/year and up to 10% in 20 years. Risk is increased with:

- duration of the UC,
- extent of UC—pancolitis has the highest risk, whereas ulcerative proctitis has no increased risk, and
- continuous inflammation.

Any patient who has had UC for 10 years should have a colonoscopy with biopsy to check for dysplasia. Once started, normal colonoscopic screening for cancer is every 1–3 years.

Treatment of UC

UC is cured with surgery! But it may be difficult surgery, so reserve it for findings of cancer or dysplasia! Complete colectomy is recommended for patients with dysplasia in a mass lesion and for high-grade dysplasia in flat mucosa. Repeat colonoscopy in 6 months if there is low-grade dysplasia without inflammation. Some authorities recommend colectomy if low-grade dysplasia without inflammation is confirmed on 2 biopsies within 6 months. Repeat in 6–12 months for dysplasia with inflammation (usually not precancerous).

Table 1-3: Tx of Inflammatory Bowel Disease. Comparison of Treatments Used in Ulcerative Colitis and Crohn Disease

ULCERATIVE COLITIS

SEVERITY:		MILD	MODERATE	SEVERE		FULMINANT	REMISSION
... definition of severity	Stools/d	< 4	Between mild and severe	> 6		> 10	Normal
	KUB	Normal		Air, edema, thumbprinting		Bowel dilation	
	Physical exam	Normal; but h/o intermittent fecal blood		Fever, Abd tenderness, freq fecal blood		Fever, Abd tenderness, and distention	
TREATMENT:		Distal disease: Rectal corticosteroids; oral or rectal aminosalicylates Extensive colon involvement: Oral aminosalicylates		Distal disease: Oral or rectal corticosteroids Extensive colon involvement: Oral corticosteroids		IV corticosteroids IV cyclosporine or infliximab if resistant to corticosteroids	Oral aminosalicylates (rectal okay if distal disease) Oral azathioprine or mercaptopurine if steroid dependent or refractory

CROHN DISEASE

SEVERITY: Definitions same as for UC	MILD	MODERATE	SEVERE/FULMINANT	POST-OP	REMISSION
TREATMENT:	Oral amino-salycilates; Metronidazole	Oral corticosteroids; Azathioprine, 6-MP, or methotrexate if steroid depdt or refractory	IV corticosteroids; IV infliximab; Elemental diet or TPN = transient benefit	Metronidazole (delays anastomotic recurrence - danger of neuropathy)	Oral aminosalicylate; Azathioprine or 6-MP especially if steroid dependent or refractory; Note: 6-MP is now standard maintenance therapy

Note the differences and similarities in these treatments! Metronidazole and diet (bowel rest) are ineffective in UC. Rectal preparations are used only in UC of the distal colon

notes

Other indications for UC surgery besides cancer are:
- intractable disease
- growth retardation in children
- exsanguinating hemorrhage
- complication from therapy
- perforation
- toxic megacolon
- steroid dependence
- stricture

[Know all the treatment.] Therapy for UC is changing due to the advent of 5-ASA compounds without sulfa, as well as the addition of corticosteroids. UC, as a more acute inflammatory process, responds to steroids much better than CD. See Table 1-3.

For mild disease, there are several options. Oral sulfasalazine, oral mesalamine, rectal mesalamine (suppository for proctitis; enema for proctosigmoiditis), and hydrocortisone enemas. All have similar efficacy—75% response and 30% remission after 2 months. The HC enemas have few side effects and give quicker symptom relief than mesalamine.

For moderate-to-severe UC, initial therapy is oral prednisone. Hospitalize patients with fulminant UC and treat with IV corticosteroids; the patient may need a colectomy if the fulminant symptoms persist for > 48 hours.

Maintenance therapy after remission:
- Sulfasalazine, mesalamine, or olsalazine daily for 1–2 years.
- Azathioprine and 6-mercaptopurine for frequent recurrences/steroid dependence; treatment may take 3–4 months to show an effect.
- Cyclosporine provides short-term remission in 40–50% of patients with severe colitis, but long-term remission in only 20–30%.

A few buzzwords: Tenesmus (UC); Rectal bleeding (UC); Fecal soiling (think fistula = CD); Hydronephrosis without stones (obstruction from inflammatory mass = CD); Pneumaturia (think fistula to the bladder = CD).

DIARRHEA

OVERVIEW

Diarrhea is defined variably as > 200–250 gm/day of stool. Average daily output is 150–180 gm. Note: Small-volume, loose stools are not considered diarrhea.

Diarrhea is typically categorized by duration of symptoms. Acute is < 2 weeks, persistent is 2–4 weeks, and chronic is > 1 month.

ACUTE DIARRHEA

The infectious causes of acute diarrhea are covered in the ID section under Common ID Syndromes: Gastrointestinal.

Introduction

Acute diarrhea is usually of an infectious etiology, but it may also be caused by food poisoning or drug side effects.

Diagnosis of Acute Diarrhea

Do the simple things first! Check diet history. Lab: First check fecal WBC—if elevated, do C+S, O+P (O+P especially if positive travel history), and +/- sigmoidoscopy with biopsy. If you suspect E. coli O157:H7 (enterohemorrhagic E. coli – EHEC), specifically ask for MacConkey-sorbitol agar for the stool culture media. If you suspect Clostridium difficile, also add C. difficile toxin assay.

Rectal/colonic biopsies can be useful in differentiating infectious colitis from inflammatory bowel disease. Crypt abscesses may be found in both, but crypt distortions are found only in inflammatory bowel disease.

Treatment of Acute Diarrhea

Generally, invasive diarrhea is treated with TMP/SMX, but use macrolides for Campylobacter and metronidazole for amebiasis. Antibiotics may prolong Salmonella infections and therefore are usually not used. Quinolones (especially ciprofloxacin) are effective in all of these, except Campylobacter (resistance by Campylobacter to quinolones is too high to use them empirically) and amebiasis, and are an alternative first choice.

Another big exception is E. coli O157:H7 infection (EHEC), which is treated only symptomatically. Antibiotics are contraindicated!

Now, go to the ID section to review more detail on the specific organisms and treatments!

CHRONIC DIARRHEA

Mechanisms

Overview

Again, chronic diarrhea is loose stools > 200–250 gm per day for > 1 month.

Chronic diarrhea can be classified according to 3 mechanisms: osmotic, secretory, and increased motility. First, we will compare and contrast osmotic and secretory mechanisms (note that "[x]" means "concentration of x").

Normal: In all normal bowel contents, the number of cations $[Na^+]$ plus $[K^+]$ are equal to the anions: $[Cl^-]$ + $[HCO_3^-]$ plus other absorbable anions (mostly short-chained fatty acids that should be absorbed early in bowel transit).

Therefore, calculated stool osmolality can be said to be = $2[Na^+ + K^+]$ which = serum osmolality which is typically 280–300 mOsm/L—or, for the equations, 290 mOsm/L.

Note that stool total osmolality = serum osmolality is true for all types of diarrhea.

Because the fluid in secretory diarrhea is, in essence, an ultrafiltrate of the serum, secretory diarrhea is similar to normal stool in that $2[Na^+ + K^+] = 290$ mOsm/L, whereas in osmotic

notes

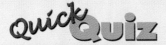
diarrhea, part of the osmolality is due to unmeasured, nonabsorbable, osmotically active molecules—so the $2[Na^+ + K^+]$ is much less than 290 mOsm/L. This difference is usually > 50 mOsm/L.

Secretory Diarrhea

In secretory diarrhea, $2[Na^+ + K^+]$ of the stool = 290 mOsm/L (i.e., measured serum osmolality). There is more stool volume in secretory diarrhea than in osmotic diarrhea, often > 1 L/d, so there is obviously an increased secretion of electrolytes; thus the patient is at risk for an electrolyte deficiency. There are many causes of secretory diarrhea:

- enterotoxins from *E. coli*, cholera, and *S. aureus*
- villous adenomas
- gastrinomas
- VIPomas that produce vasoactive intestinal peptide (VIP)
- microscopic colitis
- collagenous colitis
- bile acids

Table 1-4: Osmotic vs Secretory Diarrhea		
	Osmotic	Secretory
Volume /day	< 1 L	> 1 L
Effect of Fasting on Diarrhea	Decreases > 50%	Decreases < 20%
Serum (= Total Stool) Osmolality	290	290
Example [Na⁺] Example [K⁺] So [Na⁺] + [K⁺] =	40 20 60	105 40 145
2([Na⁺] + [K⁺])	120	290
Osmotic Gap	> 50	< 50

A 24–48 hour fast does not stop secretory diarrhea, except in fatty acid- and bile acid-related diarrheas.
See Table 1-4.

Osmotic Diarrhea

In osmotic diarrhea, ([serum osmolality] $- 2[Na^+ + K^+]$) > 50. So, there is at least a 50 mOsm/L osmotic gap that is due to a nonabsorbable osmotic agent. A 24-hour fast does resolve the diarrhea. Lactase deficiency is one of the most common causes of osmotic diarrhea. Other common causes are: Mg-containing laxatives and antacids, non- or poorly absorbable carbohydrates (xylitol, lactulose, sorbitol, fructose), and nutrient malabsorption (i.e., pancreatic insufficiency, celiac disease, bacterial overgrowth). If an osmotic diarrhea persists despite a 24-hour fast, suspect surreptitious ingestion of a Mg-containing antacid. Most laxatives, including castor oil, cause an osmotic diarrhea.

Note: Stool osmolality that is greater than serum osmolality indicates an improper stool collection procedure.

Diarrhea 2° Increased Motility

Increased motility: The last mechanism of diarrhea is increased motility. The dysmotility syndromes include antibiotic-associated diarrhea, hyperthyroidism, carcinoid, and irritable bowel. Erythromycin is one of the most common causes of antibiotic-associated diarrhea. It binds to motilin receptors, thereby increasing bowel motility. Treatment for most antibiotic-associated diarrhea is to stop the drug. Antibiotic-associated colitis is a different animal (*C. difficile*, discussed later).

Different mechanisms of diarrhea may occur together in certain diseases. In celiac disease, osmotic and secretory mechanisms coexist because there is malabsorption of carbohydrates (osmotic) and fat (secretory). Exudative diarrhea (i.e., high fecal WBCs; includes invasive bacteria and IBD) contains all 3 mechanisms: Inflammation causes altered motility, and malabsorption can cause both osmotic and secretory components.

Chronic, secretory diarrhea has a high volume (> 1 L/day despite fasting), few (if any) fecal WBCs, and fecal $2[Na^+ + K^+]$ is approximately equal to the serum osmolality. Etiology: secretory tumors (e.g., villous adenomas), (low) bile acid-related diarrhea, and steatorrhea.

Special Note: Laxative abuse leads to osmotic diarrhea with an osmotic gap > 50.

Classification of chronic diarrhea by mechanism is discussed in the next topic.

Causes of Chronic Diarrhea

AIDS

[Know!]: 60% of AIDS patients have diarrhea and weight loss. If the patient with AIDS has diarrhea and weight loss without fever, suspect *Cryptosporidia* (usual cause), *E. histolytica*, *Giardia*, *Isospora*, *Strongyloides*, and AIDS enteropathy. All of these organisms are noninvasive. With fever, think *Myco-*

bacterium, *Campylobacter*, *Salmonella*, *Cryptococcus*, *Histoplasma*, and CMV (these are covered in the ID section under Common ID Syndromes: Gastrointestinal).

Volume is a big clue in AIDS-associated diarrhea. > 1 L/day suggests a small bowel cause.

A CD4 count < 200, especially if accompanied by weight loss, points to an infectious etiology rather than AIDS enteropathy.

IBD

[Know!]: Chronic inflammatory diseases of the colon (UC and Crohn colitis) cause loose stools with many WBCs and histologic damage. Volume may be greater or less than 200 gm/day. Chronic, bloody stools suggests UC. Chronic loose stools associated with chronic RLQ abdominal cramping, especially palpation of thickened bowel in the RLQ, suggests CD. Note: Fecal WBCs and blood are found in both invasive diarrhea and UC. See pg 1-15 for more on IBD.

Diabetes

Diabetic diarrhea may be caused by:
- use of dietetic foods rich in sorbitol (erroneously labeled "sugarless"),
- visceral autonomic neuropathy (especially suspect this in the incontinent diabetic patient), and
- malabsorption (less common) due to sprue (present in 5% of diabetics), pancreatic insufficiency, or bacterial overgrowth (treat with metronidazole or amoxicillin-clavulanate).

Carbohydrate Intolerance

Consider carbohydrate intolerance in all patients with chronic diarrhea who excessively ingest beverages rich in sorbitol and fructose. Note: Coke/Pepsi has 40 gm of fructose per 16 oz (480 mL).

Carcinoid

Carcinoid [Know!] is a less common cause of chronic diarrhea. Most carcinoids are asymptomatic and nonsecreting. Most nonsecreting carcinoids are found in the appendix. About 75% of the secreting, symptomatic carcinoids are in the ileum. Gastric carcinoids are related to hypergastrinemic states (this aspect is discussed on pg 1-13).

The symptomatic carcinoids [Know] secrete various vasoactive mediators, including 5-hydroxytryptophan, 5-hydroxytryptamine, and histamine, which cause paroxysmal flushing; crampy, explosive diarrhea, and sometimes tachycardia and hypotension. The flushing is often bright red with well-defined borders and can be on the whole body—including hands and soles. Because tryptophan, a precursor of niacin, is used up in carcinoid syndrome, niacin deficiency may occur.

Carcinoids that cause the diarrhea have already metastasized to the liver—and can be seen on CT/MRI of the liver!

The bronchial carcinoids (rare) cause more dramatic symptoms than the intestinal secreting type because bronchial carcinoids dump the vasoactive mediators directly into the arterial circulation.

Diagnosis: Check 24-hour urine for 5-hydroxyindoleacetic acid (5-HIAA)—a breakdown product of 5-hydroxytryptamine. Normal is < 10 mg/24 hr; with carcinoid, patient has > 25 mg/24 hr. CT of liver should show metastatic lesions.

Visceral Autonomic Neuropathy

Visceral autonomic neuropathy is characterized by:
- delayed gastric emptying (i.e., gastroparesis),
- postural decrease in blood pressure,
- anhidrosis (inability to tolerate heat, lack of functioning sweat glands)—especially in lower extremities,
- fecal incontinence,
- impotence (men), and
- urinary overflow incontinence.

Microscopic Colitis

Microscopic colitis consists of both collagenous colitis and lymphocytic colitis. These patients have normal-looking mucosa but abnormal findings on mucosa biopsy (hence the name microscopic colitis). These patients have a chronic secretory, watery diarrhea.

Colonoscopy is normal, but wall biopsy of the normal looking mucosa shows a lymphocytic infiltrate or a collagenous band in the submucosa. Know that these entities do not progress to IBD.

Other

Other causes of chronic diarrhea include:
- steatorrhea (discussed further below),
- endocrinopathies (hyper- & hypothyroidism, adrenal insufficiency),
- colon cancer,
- radiation-induced disease, and
- fecal incontinence (radiation; diabetes; rectal surgery; and childbirth injury to anal sphincter, especially forceps delivery).

Patients do not want to mention "fecal incontinence." They frequently will get around the issue by asking "for medication to control the diarrhea." Ask patients with diarrhea if they experience fecal incontinence more than once a week. If so, the differential diagnosis includes the items listed above.

Chronic Loose Stools

The following may cause loose stools < 200 gm/day, so do not meet the criteria of diarrhea:

Lactase deficiency (lactose intolerance) is a common cause of loose stools, although the volume is usually < 200 gm/day.

Irritable bowel syndrome (IBS) has loose stools with normal daily volume. See pg 1-26 for more on IBS.

notes

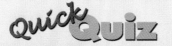
Diagnosis of Chronic Diarrhea

Note: As soon as you make the diagnosis of chronic diarrhea, stop testing.

Stage 1: Stool O&P & fecal leukocytes x 3.
Stool pH. *C. difficile* toxin assay. Weight of stool/24 hours. 3-day fecal fat (or if Sudan stain is positive, do the fecal fat). Also chem 20, thyroid profile, and gastrin level. Lactose-free diet if lactase deficiency is at all suggested by history.

Stage 2: Immunoabsorbent assay for giardiasis.
If steatorrhea is confirmed, order KUB for pancreatic calcification (discussed in detail shortly). If diabetic has suggestive history: Do either a 14C-glycocholate breath test for bacterial overgrowth or (more often) just treat empirically. If > 1000 cc/d of stool, check vasoactive intestinal polypeptide. Also may do sigmoidoscopy and high-quality UGI.

Check for laxative abuse by:
• specific urine tests for bisacodyl, anthraquinones, and phenolphthalein,
• stool osmotic gap > 100 mOsm/L (magnesium-containing), and
• stool measurement of phosphate and sulfate.
If the stool osmolality is low, the patient could be adding water or urine to the stool

Stage 3: EGD and colonoscopy.
A significant number of patients have no discernible cause of the diarrhea and have no abdominal pain and normal EGD and colonoscopy. These patients have idiopathic chronic diarrhea. Often, a hospital stay is required after stage 3 to redo the previous tests with better controls.

Loose Stools and Fecal Impaction

Watery stool will leak around a fecal impaction, causing small-volume watery effluent. See more on fecal impaction on pg 1-34.

MALABSORPTION

Overview

Malabsorption may be short-lived, but patients often present with a chronic diarrhea. Malabsorption can be caused by:
• decreased small bowel mucosal transport, and
• decreased digestion.
The "Big 6" lab tests are those done in the routine workup for malabsorption. These look for:
Low: albumin, Ca^{++}, cholesterol, carotene, serum iron, and Prolonged PTT. These are discussed a little later in this section but first we will discuss the causes of malabsorption—which can be divided into decreased mucosal transport (something wrong with intestinal uptake) or decreased digestion (not enough digestive enzymes).

Malabsorption Due to Decreased Mucosal Transport

Introduction

Decreased mucosal transport: May be caused by celiac disease, tropical sprue, common variable immune deficiency with hypogammaglobulinemia, Whipple disease, intestinal lymphoma, eosinophilic gastroenteritis, bacterial overgrowth, and other small bowel disease. These are discussed below.

Celiac disease

Celiac disease (gluten-sensitive enteropathy, previously celiac sprue, nontropical sprue) is an amazingly common disease considering how infrequently it is diagnosed. It occurs in up to 1% of the population of most countries. Gluten is contained in wheat, barley, and rye.
Celiac disease is an autoimmune intestinal disorder in which there is a toxic reaction with dietary gluten resulting in small bowel villous atrophy and crypt hypertrophy with resulting malabsorption. It is prevalent in Ireland, can cause growth retardation, and is associated with HLA-DQ2 and HLA-DQ8. It may go into remission during adolescence, then recur.

Extraintestinal manifestations are:
• iron deficiency anemia (most common presentation; iron is absorbed mostly in the duodenum), low Hgb, MCV, and ferritin; the only condition that decreases ferritin is Fe deficiency;
• abnormal serum aminotransferases;
• dermatitis herpetiformis – discussed below;
• osteoporosis;
• osteomalacia;
• neuropsychiatric symptoms; and
• dental enamel defects.

notes

Primary intestinal lymphoma is a rare, late complication of celiac disease. If detected early, the patient may have mild symptoms like bloating and loose stools.

Associated deficiencies. Know:
- iron
- folic acid
- calcium
- vitamin D
- vitamin B_{12} (rarely)

There is a wide spectrum of presentations. Patients often have little or no GI symptoms and may present with only a psychiatric disorder or osteomalacia or a purulent pustular rash.

Dermatitis herpetiformis is a manifestation of celiac disease in which there are vesiculopapular eruptions on the face, trunk, buttocks, sacrum and extensor surfaces of elbows and knees.

Most patients with dermatitis herpetiformis do not have abdominal symptoms, although 85% have the characteristic findings on intestinal wall biopsy.

Diagnosis of celiac disease has the following 4 requirements:
1) evidence of malabsorption (steatorrhea, weight loss)
2) abnormal small bowel biopsy
3) usually (but not necessarily) a positive antiendomysial antibody or tissue transglutaminase antibody test
4) a positive response to a gluten-free diet (clinical, chemical, and histological)

More on antibody tests. The best are:
- IgA antiendomysial Ab and
- tissue transglutaminase (tTG) antibody.

Antigliadin antibodies (AGA) are sensitive but not specific and are superseded by antiendomysial Ab and tTG Ab. Since IgA deficiency occurs in 1–2% of U.S. population, if antiendomysial antibody is negative with strong suspicion of sprue, check serum IgA levels. These antibody tests may also be useful for determining latent celiac disease, or as a measure of compliance with the gluten-free diet.

Note: The small bowel biopsy results are characteristic but not pathognomonic, since you may see similar villous atrophy with hypogammaglobulinemia ("hypogammaglobulinemic sprue"), small intestinal bacterial overgrowth, lactose intolerance, giardiasis, peptic duodenitis, and tropical sprue! Many small bowel disease processes can cause villous atrophy.

Treat celiac disease with a gluten-free diet (GFD) +/- initial corticosteroids. 80% eventually respond to a GFD, although it may take awhile. For those patients not responding to a GFD, consider:
- noncompliance
- intestinal lymphoma
- microscopic colitis
- T-cell enteropathy
- pancreatic insufficiency
- collagenous sprue (see below)
- ulcerative jejunoileitis
- lactose intolerance 2° lactase deficiency (damaged mucosa)

Now that you know about celiac disease, what test will you remember to order in a patient presenting with the following problems?
A 16-year-old presents with a diagnosis of bipolar disorder.
A 33-year-old presents with bone pain in his spine and legs.
A 28-year-old presents with a purulent papulovesicular eruption on her extensor elbows and knees.
A 30-year-old presents with anemia and heme-negative stool, low Hgb, MCV, and serum ferritin.
Good! Antibody test for celiac disease. Celiac disease is a commonly missed diagnosis.

Collagenous Sprue

Collagenous sprue is an unusual possible variant of celiac disease in which the small bowel biopsy shows flattened mucosa with large masses of subepithelial eosinophilic hyaline material in the lamina propria. ~ 30% of those with celiac disease have some collagen deposition, and 8% have dense deposition. More collagen deposition probably indicates worse prognosis.

Tropical Sprue

Tropical sprue: causes malabsorption with partial villous atrophy that is probably of an infectious etiology. It is endemic in areas of the Caribbean, S. Africa, Venezuela, India, and S.E. Asia (i.e., the equatorial areas). Patients often have megaloblastic anemia.

Treatment: tetracycline or TMP/SMX for 3–6 months. Folic acid replacement can also be effective either alone or as adjunctive treatment.

Whipple Disease

Whipple disease is caused by *Tropheryma whippelii*, a Gram-positive actinomycete. The cardinal tetrad of symptoms is:
1) arthralgias—the most common symptom preceding diagnosis! (much more so than abdominal problems!);
2) abdominal pain;
3) weight loss; and
4) diarrhea.

Patients may have severe malabsorption—often with marked hypoalbuminemia and neurologic symptoms. Some of these symptoms are the result of lymphatic obstruction.

Upper endoscopy with small intestine biopsy is the diagnostic procedure of choice. Small bowel biopsy shows specific foamy macrophages and is positive for PAS staining bacterial remnants. You can also check CSF for *T. whippelii* by PCR, which is diagnostic if found.

Treat with ceftriaxone or PCN for 14 days and then treat for 1 year with TMP/SMX. [Know: Relapse often manifests with CNS symptoms.]

DDx: These symptoms also may be caused by lymphatic blockage from primary intestinal (or other) lymphoma.

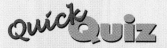

Eosinophilic Gastroenteritis

Eosinophilic gastroenteritis can mimic intestinal lymphoma and regional enteritis. Patients have N/V/diarrhea, abdominal pain, weight loss, albumin wasting, and iron deficiency anemia. They often have a peripheral eosinophilia, and even though it is thought to be due to an allergy to certain foods—which would be mediated by IgE—only 20% have specific food allergies with an increased IgE.

Treat with corticosteroids and avoidance of the causative foods. *Strongyloides* can also cause a peripheral eosinophilia (*Giardia* does not), so be sure to rule this out before you start the steroids!

Short Bowel Syndrome

Short bowel syndrome occurs after massive resection of the small bowel, usually due to:
• severe ischemic injury or
• surgery for small bowel volvulus, jejunoileal bypass for morbid obesity, or multiple surgeries for Crohn disease.

Short bowel syndrome is likely when there is (roughly) < 2 feet (60 cm) of small bowel—especially when the proximal jejunum and/or distal ileum are involved. Lifelong TPN is likely if the remaining small bowel is < 100 cm and there is loss of ileocecal valve.

These patients are susceptible to calcium oxalate kidney stones (2° steatorrhea) and gastric acid hypersecretion.

Treat with a low-fat diet and vitamin supplements. TPN may be needed after large resection while waiting for bowel adaptation.

Malabsorption Due to Decreased Digestion

Overview

Two main causes of decreased digestion:

1) Pancreatic insufficiency: as can be seen in chronic pancreatitis, pancreatic cancer, and cystic fibrosis. Determine pancreatic insufficiency by the qualitative stool exam, revealing undigested muscle fibers, neural fat, split fat, and low levels of fecal elastase.

The undigested muscle fibers indicate impaired digestion. Low fecal elastase is characteristic of pancreatogenous steatorrhea.

Further confirm impaired digestion by a positive response to treatment with pancreatic enzymes. The xylose absorption test may also be done during the workup (discussed below), and is normal.

You must rule out pancreatic cancer if there is evidence of pancreatic insufficiency in patients > 55 years old.

2) Bile acid deficiency: a) Ileal resection (> 100 cm—see below) or disease that decreases bile acid uptake; b) Severe liver disease, which decreases production of bile acids; c) Zollinger-Ellison syndrome (ZES), in which the patient has increased acidity in the small bowel that precipitates the bile acids; d) Bacterial overgrowth resulting in the breakdown of bile acids, making them useless for fat digestion (discussed below).

• Steatorrhea is the best indicator of malabsorption (of any type) because it usually is the most prominent problem.
• Sudan stain of the stool (for fat) is the best screening test. Serum carotene levels are a less specific indicator for malabsorption (see next).
• The 3-day, quantitative fecal fat measurement is the "gold standard" for determining steatorrhea. Because diarrhea itself can cause up to 14 gm/d fecal fat, steatorrhea is defined as > 14 gm/d of fecal fat.

Steatorrhea from pancreatic insufficiency causes the most fecal fat (can be > 50 gm/d). Any patient having > 40 gm/d of fecal fat almost certainly has pancreatic insufficiency—barring history of intestinal resection, which can also increase fecal fat to these levels.

Diagnosing the Cause: Transport vs. Digestion

Diagnosing etiology of the malabsorption: First, determine whether it is a small bowel mucosal problem or pancreatic insufficiency (transport vs. digestion), by using the xylose (D-xylose) absorption test. D-xylose requires normal transmucosal transport, but it does not require digestion by pancreatic enzymes to be absorbed.

[Know!]: A normal xylose absorption test result (> 4.5 gm of a 25 gm oral dose excreted in the urine over 5 hr, or patient has a > 20 mg/dL serum level) in a patient with steatorrhea excludes diffuse, small bowel disease (i.e., CD, short bowel syndrome) and makes pancreatic insufficiency more likely.

notes

These patients are often empirically treated with pancreatic enzymes. Resolution of the symptoms is both therapeutic and confirms the diagnosis. Note: Normal urinary xylose after a 25 gm oral load is 6.0 +/- 1.5 gm over 5 hr.

On the other hand, a low result (< 5 gm) can be caused not only by small bowel disease, but also by many other conditions, including poor gastric emptying, bacterial overgrowth, ascites, renal insufficiency, and old age! But, if the patient definitely has steatorrhea, the likelihood is that the diagnosis is small bowel disease since most of the other causes of an abnormal xylose test do not cause steatorrhea. So, xylose test low? Do a small bowel biopsy!

Again, normal D-xylose = normal small bowel.

The absorption of carotene, vitamin K, vitamin D, folate, and iron are also, like xylose, independent of pancreatic enzyme digestion. So chronic, non-bloody diarrhea with low serum carotene, hypocalcemia, hypoprothrombinemia, and/or Fe deficiency anemia suggests a small bowel malabsorption problem rather than a pancreatic disorder—this is true only if the patient has a normal dietary intake and only after prolonged disease. Conversely, chronic diarrhea and normal levels of the above indicates pancreatic insufficiency. An alcoholic who has an elevated prothrombin time easily corrected by vitamin K more likely has malabsorption as the cause of the high PT—not liver disease!

Summary: This is really easy! Malabsorption (steatorrhea)—
- Low "anything" suggests small bowel mucosal problem or bacterial overgrowth.
- Normal xylose absorption test (i.e., carotene, calcium, and others also normal) suggests pancreatic insufficiency—especially if there is very high fecal fat.

Bacterial Overgrowth

There can be combined causes of malabsorption, as in bacterial overgrowth, which results in bile acid deconjugation and variable patchy destruction of intestinal villi.

Patients with bacterial overgrowth usually have moderate steatorrhea, but that may not be their presenting complaint. The overgrowth of bacteria makes more folate but decreases absorption of B_{12}, so you can get the odd finding of macrocytosis with high folate and low B_{12} levels.

Bacterial overgrowth occurs in a variety of conditions:
- structural abnormalities—diverticula, fistulae, strictures, after ileocecal resection
- motility disorders—peristalsis is a major mechanism for clearing the small intestine of bacteria (may be defective in diabetes and scleroderma)
- achlorhydria—acid in the stomach kills bacteria before it enters the small bowel
- immune disorders—immunoglobulins secreted in small bowel may decrease bacterial growth

Diagnose bacterial overgrowth with the lactulose breath test and sometimes the C14-glycocholate breath test. Also remember the high folate levels with low B_{12} and microcytosis. CT or UGI will show any small bowel diverticula (usually from scleroderma) and dilated small bowel.

The specific overgrowth tests are usually available only at large medical centers. Bacterial overgrowth is often treated empirically with antibiotics after suggestive history and lab findings. Usually 2 antibiotics (most commonly, amoxicillin-clavulanic acid + metronidazole) that cover anaerobes and aerobes.

Bowel Resection and Diarrhea

Massive resection of small bowel: Causes malabsorption (short bowel syndrome), especially if the terminal ileum and ileocecal valve are resected.
- \> 100 cm of terminal ileum resected: Malabsorption due to decreased bile acids. See under Crohn Disease, Terminal Ileum Problems on pg 1-17.
- < 100 cm of terminal ileum resected: Bile acid-induced diarrhea from bile acids not resorbed in the terminal ileum, and entering the colon.

IRRITABLE BOWEL SYNDROME

OVERVIEW

A large part of a gastroenterologist's practice consists of functional complaints. ~ 15% of the population has signs/symptoms of irritable bowel syndrome (IBS), and, by far, women make up the majority of cases. IBS has characteristic symptoms of frequent, small stools with mucus, and abdominal pain relieved by defecation. These symptoms may be either continuous or recurring. There are no nocturnal or organic symptoms. Patients generally have an increased bowel motor response to emotional and physical stimuli, but these motor patterns are not specific to IBS. Patients with IBS are more likely to have been abused in childhood.

DIAGNOSIS OF IBS

Establish diagnosis of IBS by:
1) excluding other diseases and
2) looking for characteristic symptoms.

Only rarely do cases need invasive evaluation with colonoscopy or sigmoidoscopy.

These patients are more likely to have psychosocial dysfunction that doesn't meet criteria for major disorders. They may have neuroses, anxiety, or depression. They are also more likely to have a history of physical or sexual abuse.

1) Excluding other diseases:
Celiac disease: 2–4% of IBS patients, especially those referred to a secondary center, have celiac disease (pg 1-23), which can be screened out with antiendomysial Ab or tissue transglutaminase Ab.

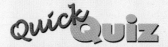
Lactose intolerance: Rule out lactose intolerance. Also consider that 33% of patients with lactose intolerance do not improve on a lactose-restricted diet because they have concurrent IBS!

Sorbitol: Rule out excessive sorbitol use (in sugarless candies).

2) Looking for characteristic symptoms:

The characteristic symptom pattern of abdominal pain and changed bowel habits has been formalized into the International Classification for Irritable Bowel Syndrome—usually called the Rome criteria. These are [Know]:

At least 3 months of continuous or recurrent:
- abdominal pain relieved by defecation or accompanied by a change in frequency or consistency of stool,
    and
- disturbed defecation at least 25% of the time, consisting of 2 or more:
    - altered frequency
    - passage of mucus
    - abdominal distention
    - altered consistency
    - altered stool passage
    and
- no constitutional signs or symptoms, such as fever, weight loss, anorexia, and anemia. Specifically, no nocturnal symptoms!

TREATMENT OF IBS

Reassurance is paramount, as shown by the very impressive 60–70% (!) response to placebo by these patients—although only 30% have adequate relief with placebo. It is critical to form a therapeutic physician-patient relationship.

Behavioral and cognitive therapies help the psychosocial issues.

Fiber supplementation is a traditional standard of care, although not proven to be effective.

Probiotics such as *Lactobacillus acidophilus* and *Bifidobacterium longum* can be tried.

Antispasmodic agents used for IBS are anticholinergics (dicyclomine, hyoscyamine) and have more side effects than benefits long-term. Okay for short-term or intermittent use.

Tricyclic antidepressants (TCA) in low doses work well for IBS, especially if they have loose stools, because TCAs slow bowel motility and may improve any neuropathic pain.

Motility drugs: Loperamide decreases motility and increases sphincter tone and is good with loose stools.

Lubiprostone (Amitiza®) is effective for constipation-predominant IBS.

5-hydroxytryptomin (serotonin) 3 receptor antagonists have had problems with side effects (ischemic colitis and severe constipation). Alosetron was pulled from the market and now is back, but under strict FDA control. Other agents include ondansetron and granisetron.

5-hydroxytryptomin (serotonin) 4 receptor agonists have had even more issues (cardiac side effects!), and the only agent in this class—tegaserod—was pulled by the FDA in March 2007. It is now back, under investigational use.

COLON CANCER

OVERVIEW

Colon cancer risk factors:
- age > 50
- ulcerative colitis
- BRCA1 mutation
- obesity
- history of adenomatous polyps
- Crohn colitis
- acromegaly
- smoking
- 1st degree relatives with colon cancer or adenomatous polyps
- familial polyposis (FP) syndromes (see next)
- diets high in calories and animal fat
- hereditary, nonpolyposis colon cancer (HNPCC—see below)

Lifetime risk of colon cancer is 4%.

Diagnostic flags for colon cancer:
- anorexia
- weight loss
- anemia
- fever
- heme+ stools
- nocturnal stools
- onset of symptoms after age 45

Also remember: Endocarditis caused by either *Strep bovis* or *Clostridium septicus* is often associated with colon cancer, so conduct a thorough GI workup in these patients.

Low-dose aspirin (81 mg) appears to have a mild preventative effect on the development of recurrent colon adenomas, but low-dose aspirin alone is not enough to decrease colon cancer risk. Full-dose aspirin is necessary for reducing risk of colon cancer. Protective effect of aspirin is related to:
- dose of aspirin,
- frequency of use per week, and
- duration of use (years).

Most GI cancers arise from adenomas. 25% of colorectal cancers are located beyond the splenic flexure.

notes

Table 1-5: Malignant Potential vs Size			
	< 1 cm	1-2 cm	> 2 cm
Tubular	1%	10%	34%
Mixed (TV)	4%	9%	45%
Villous	10%	10%	54%

Adenomas with "advanced" features are defined as:
- > 1 cm (see Table 1-5, 10-fold increase from < 1 cm to > 1 cm with tubular polyps) and
- histology is villous or tubulovillous. (Note: just tubular is usually benign—especially if < 1 cm.)

"Advanced" means likely to develop into cancer. Progression to cancer from an early adenoma takes 5–10 years. Diet plays a role in GI cancer—possible dietary factors include high animal protein and fats, low fiber, and low calcium. Be sure and discuss these important considerations with patients on a "low-carb" diet!

Again, large or villous adenomatous polyps are likely to harbor or progress to cancer.

Perspective: ~ 30% of people > 40 years old have adenomatous polyps, but only 1% of adenomatous polyps ever become malignant.

Hyperplastic polyps have no malignant potential and contain no features of dysplasia. This makes sense because hyperplasia, by definition, is increased growth of normal tissue.

After polyps are found, follow-up depends on the type of polyp, size, number found, and family history. Only adenomatous polyps require specific follow-up. Hyperplastic polyps (except for those with a hyperplastic polyposis syndrome) have same followup as no polyp (10 years). The 2008 American Cancer Society guidelines recommend the following:

- Patients with 1 or 2 small tubular adenomas with low-grade dysplasia should have repeat colonoscopy 5–10 years after initial polypectomy.

- Patients with 3–10 adenomas or 1 adenoma > 1 cm or any adenoma with villous features or high-grade dysplasia should have repeat colonoscopy in 3 years.

- Patients with > 10 adenomas should have repeat colonoscopy < 3 years (consider the possibility of an underlying familial syndrome—see below)

- Patients with sessile adenomas that are removed piecemeal require repeat colonoscopy in 2–6 months to verify complete removal.

FAMILIAL POLYPOSIS SYNDROMES

Overview

Colon Cancer Families: Polyposis vs. Nonpolyposis syndromes.

Familial Polyposis Syndromes

The familial (or hereditary) polyposis syndromes are all autosomal dominant (AD). In order of decreasing cancer potential:

1) Familial adenomatous polyposis (FAP)—hundreds of adenomas in the colon—100% risk of cancer if not treated. These patients require a proctocolectomy by age 20! They can also get some duodenal adenomas, which also have a high risk of cancer. After colectomy, patients with FAP tend to next get duodenal cancer. They are also at increased risk of developing secondary tumors (ampullary adenomas, cancers). Giant stomach tumors are common in FAP patients, but they are benign.

2) Gardner syndrome—a variant of FAP with more extraintestinal benign growths. The adenomas have the same risk of cancer as FAP (100%). These patients often have bone lesions (osteomas) and soft tissue tumors. Treatment is the same as FAP. Question: Patient has multiple osteomas found incidentally on an x-ray. What do you do? Colonoscopy!

3) Peutz-Jeghers syndrome—multiple hamartomatous polyps throughout the small bowel, and occasionally in the colorectum and stomach, plus melanotic pigmentation (freckles) on the lips and buccal mucosa.
   The most common presentation is with abdominal pain due to intussusception or bowel obstruction by a large polyp.
   Even though these polyps are hamartomas, there is still some risk of cancer because there are occasional adenomas that can become carcinomas. Risk of cancer is 50% by 60 years of age.

4) Juvenile polyposis also consists of hamartomas. This is the only one of these syndromes with no malignant potential. No follow-up needed.

Hereditary Nonpolyposis Colon Cancer

Affected persons in most colon cancer families do not have familial polyposis—rather the cancer arises from normal-appearing epithelium.

Hereditary nonpolyposis colon cancer (HNPCC or Lynch syndrome) can be defined as "the occurrence of colon cancer in at least three 1st degree relatives over at least 2 generations, and with at least 1 person diagnosed < age 50." These rather loose diagnostic criteria place Lynch syndrome in as many as 1 in 20 (5%) patients with colon cancer! Women in families with HNPCC often have greatly increased incidence of ovarian and endometrial cancer, as well as renal, ureteral, stomach, and biliary tree cancers.

Start screening at age 25 for HNPCC.

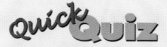

SCREENING

Review

Current screening recommendations are also covered in the General Internal Medicine section under "Screening Tests." In general, do yearly fecal occult blood testing (FOBT) in low-risk patients. Note: Yearly rectal exams are done for prostate cancer, not colorectal cancer.

The 2008 American cancer Society guidelines for colorectal cancer screening for asymptomatic adults ≥ 50 years of age has broken down the tests into the following 2 areas.

1) Tests that detect adenomatous polyps and cancer (preferred by the guideline-writing committee):
   • flexible sigmoidoscopy every 5 years, or
   • colonoscopy every 10 years, or
   • double-contrast barium enema every 5 years, or
   • CT colonography every 5 years.

2) Tests that primarily detect cancer:
   • annual guaiac-based fecal occult blood test with high test sensitivity for cancer, or
   • annual fecal immunochemical test with high test sensitivity for cancer, or

   • stool DNA test with high sensitivity for cancer, interval uncertain.

Each strategy has inherent strengths and weaknesses. FOBT is the most inexpensive and obviously least invasive, but it misses ~ 1/3 of advanced cancers. Colonoscopy has the highest yield of finding polyps and cancers, but is most costly and invasive.

If flexible sigmoidoscopy reveals a polyp, biopsy it! A full colonoscopy is then indicated if the polyp has "advanced" features, as discussed earlier: 1) any polyp > 1.0 cm or 2) histology showing villous or tubulovillous architecture.

Repeat colonoscopy every 3 years thereafter if polyp is benign. Hyperplastic is not an advanced feature; these polyps have no malignant potential.

The "10 year" rule.

Increased-risk patients: Onset of surveillance (colonoscopy) should be at age 40 years or 10 years before age at which index case is diagnosed—whichever is first.

For example: Start at age 40 if a 1st degree relative was diagnosed with an adenoma or colon cancer at age 50; start at age 20 if several 1st degree relatives had colon cancer at age 30.

Colonoscopy is the screening procedure of choice if any 1st degree relatives have had colon cancer or an adenomatous polyp, or if an adenomatous polyp has ever been found in the patient. Time between surveillance colonoscopies is dependent on the cancer potential of the polyp: see previous discussion above, under Colon Cancer Overview. Virtual colonoscopy or CT colonography is a CT scan with special software in a totally prepped patient. It has high yield for detecting larger polyps and cancers. Areas of adherent stool can be mistaken for small polyps. However, it is an excellent test for a patient who could not complete a standard colonoscopy to visualize the entirety of the colon. If abnormalities are found on CT colonography, the guidelines recommend if possible to go straight to colonoscopy, since the patient has already been prepped; otherwise the patient will have to return and do another bowel prep.

Sigmoid colon cancer can perforate the bowel wall and simulate diverticulitis. So survey for colon cancer after diverticulitis in older patients.

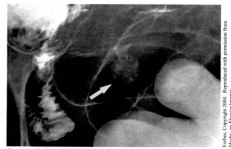

Image 1-21: Single colonic polyp on double contrast barium enema

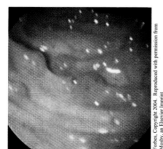

Image 1-22: Familial polyposis with multiple sessile polyps

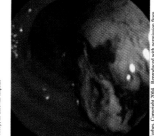

Image 1-23: Colon cancer

notes

FOBT

Fecal occult blood testing (FOBT) is positive in about 2%. This varies with age; > 5% after 60 years old. Of positive FOBTs, 2% have GI cancer.

Remember: The FOBT is negative in up to 66% of patients with colon cancer. Using 6 Hemoccult® cards (the full FOBT series) will detect advanced colonic cancer in only about 25% of patients. This makes it a pretty poor screening test, but it is used (annually or biennially) because it is quick and cheap.

Even if one FOBT is positive, do a colonoscopy. A flex-sig + ACBE (air-contrast BE) is also acceptable but less desirable.

CEA

Note: Carcinoembryonic antigen (CEA) levels are good only in checking for recurrence of colon cancer—and only if levels were elevated before surgery and reduced after surgery. CEA may also be mildly elevated in patients who smoke or who have benign biliary disease, sclerosing cholangitis, or IBD.

STAGING OF COLON CANCER

TNM Classification

The two methods for staging colon cancer are TNM and Duke's. They are similar but the TNM further classifies Stage III (Duke's stage C) into prognostically-based A, B, and C categories and, now, TNM is the preferred classification method. (Note: the 5-year survival percentages listed below are with treatment.)

The classifications with location, relative percent of occurrence, and 5-year survival with treatment are:

TNM Stage I; Duke's stage A:
• cancer confined to the mucosa and submucosa
• 23% of colon cancers
• 5-year survival is 93%

TNM Stage II; Duke's Stage B:
• cancer extending into or through the muscularis without lymph node involvement
• 31% of colon cancers
• 5-year survival to 72-85% (Stages IIB-IIA)

TNM Stage III; Duke's Stage C:
• cancer extends to the regional lymph nodes
• 26% of colon cancers
• 5-year survival is 44-64-83% (Stages IIIC-IIIB-IIIA)

TNM Stage IV; Duke's Stage D:
• distant metastases
• 20% of colon cancers
• 5-year survival is only 5%. Colon cancer virtually always metastasizes to the liver first (via portal circulation). If it involves only the rectum, the blood supply bypasses the portal circulation, and so the patient may have lung, bone, and brain mets without liver mets.

TREATMENT FOR COLON CANCER

Surgical resection is the first treatment option and is potentially curative. Recurrences after surgery are probably due to micro-metastases. Treatment for intestinal cancer consists of surgery for local excision.

The adjuvant chemotherapy consists of a 5-FU–based therapy. Typically 5-FU plus leucovorin (LV) is used. Recently trials have shown benefit from oxaliplatin being added to this regimen. This protocol is called FOLFOX.

Adjuvant chemo is effective only for Stage III or locally advanced II.

Radiation therapy prior to surgery is helpful for rectal lesions only.

Hepatic resection increases survival with solitary liver mets.

If you remove a cancerous polyp, you must do a bowel resection if the cancer extends to either a blood vessel or the cautery line.

DIVERTICULAR DISEASE AND LOWER GI BLEED

DIVERTICULAR DISEASE

Diverticular disease—4 types:
1) asymptomatic diverticulosis (most common)
2) painful diverticulosis (contraction of hypertrophied colonic muscle)
3) diverticular bleeding
4) diverticulitis

Painful diverticulosis is due to hypertrophy of both circular and longitudinal colonic musculature, which leads to luminal narrowing, pencil-thin stools, and pain before defecation. Treat with bulking agents such as psyllium (Metamucil®, Fiberall®, Serutan®, and others) and methylcellulose (Citrucel®, etc.)

Diverticular bleeding usually originates in the sigmoid colon, and usually stops spontaneously. Patients classically present with "painless maroon stool," but it can vary from black to red. Diverticular bleeding is the most common cause of colonic bleeding in the elderly; angiodysplasia is next on the

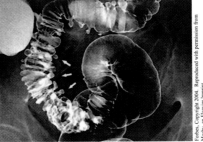
Image 1-24: Diverticular disease

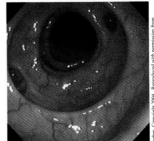
Image 1-25: Diverticular disease

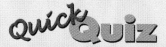

1) Are CEA levels useful for primary diagnosis, recurrence, or both in colon carcinoma? Why?

2) Surgery for cure is the rule in colon cancer. When is adjuvant chemotherapy used? When is radiation used?

3) What may be seen on abdominal CT scan in a patient with diverticulitis?

list and often results in more severe bleeds. Treatment: Stabilize patient if needed, rule out UGI bleed with NG aspirate or endoscopy. Colonoscopy only if bleeding doesn't stop.

Note: UGI bleed is suggested by a BUN/Cr ratio > 30:1, which indicates blood is being digested and its breakdown products absorbed.

Diagnose diverticular bleeding with colonoscopy or technetium-tagged RBC scan. Angiography works if bleeding is severe or continuous.

Diverticulitis is usually due to microperforations. Signs and symptoms:
- LLQ pain
- fever
- high WBC
- LLQ tenderness—may be localized, rebound tenderness
- no bleeding!

Look for signs of a sigmoid mass on physical exam, U/S, or CT. CT is most useful in assessing diverticulitis: It may show areas of thickened sigmoid colon or pericolic fluid accumulation. Avoid GI colonoscopy on any patient with diverticulitis.

Treatment of diverticulitis should cover both aerobic and anaerobic Gram-negative organisms.

Treat mild diverticulitis in a patient able to drink and without peritoneal signs with outpatient metronidazole (Gram-neg anaerobic) plus either ciprofloxacin or TMP/SMX (Gram-neg aerobic) and close follow-up.

Treatment of moderate-to-severe diverticulitis:
Inpatient parenteral treatment for those with peritoneal signs may consist of the following:
1) dual-drug therapy (best!) such as:
   aminoglycoside or ciprofloxacin (Gram-neg aerobic)
        plus
   clindamycin or metronidazole (Gram-neg anaerobic)
        or, instead of this use
2) single-drug therapy such as:
   - ticarcillin/clavulanic acid
   - imipenem/cilastatin
   - cefotetan
   - piperacillin/tazobactam
   - ampicillin/sulbactam

All these single-drug therapies cover both aerobic and anaerobic Gram-neg organisms.

Drain abscesses percutaneously.

Perforation from sigmoid colon cancer can present similarly to diverticulitis, so follow up in patients > 50 with a flex-sig/colonoscopy 4-8 weeks after the acute condition resolves.

Meckel diverticulum is the most frequent congenital GI anomaly. Although < 1/2 of these diverticula have gastric mucosa, only these ulcerate and bleed. Meckel diverticula cause 1/2 of all GI bleeds in children. It can also cause obstruction and intussusception. They may be seen with the technetium scan ("Meckel's scan"). Technetium is taken up by gastric mucosa.

ANGIODYSPLASIA AND LOWER GI BLEED

Angiodysplasia (= vascular ectasia, = AVM) is the 2nd most common cause of lower GI bleeding in the elderly (diverticular bleeding is first). Think of these as spider nevi of the GI tract.

Table 1-6: Indications for Colonoscopy
Occult bleeding
Fe deficiency anemia unless other explanation
Gross lower GI bleeding except bright red blood in a younger person
Abnormal barium enema
Adenomatous polyp – initially and for all follow-ups
History of colon cancer
1st degree relative of one with colon cancer
Familial polyposis syndromes, HNPCC/Lynch synd.
IBD: suspicion, follow-up, surveillance
Strep bovis, Clostridium septicum bacteremia
Colon ischemia (Ischemic colitis)
Persistent diarrhea with negative blood tests and not meeting criteria for diagnosis of IBS
4–8 weeks after new onset presumed diverticulitis to rule out colon cancer

Table 1-7: Use of Angiography in GI Disease
Chronic and acute mesenteric ischemia
Severe lower GI bleed
Rarely used for UGI bleed – some duodenal ulcers
TIPS in variceal bleeding
Therapeutic uses: embolization, vasopressin

notes

Bleeding in angiodysplasia may be occult to severe. Usual bleeding site is the right colon (cecum, ascending).

AVMs typically are not cauterized unless they are bleeding significantly.

Hereditary hemorrhagic telangiectasias (HHT, = Osler-Rendu-Weber) is the hereditary condition in which there are multiple AVMs affecting all the organs, including brain, lung, skin, and mucous membranes and the GI tract—especially in the upper GI tract (AVM is usually lower). Patients with HHT often have a history of epistaxis.

Endoscopic treatment can help, although there are often many lesions and not all can be treated.

COLON ISCHEMIA (ISCHEMIC COLITIS)

Colon ischemia (CI; ischemic colitis) is associated with abdominal pain (from the ischemia) and maroon stools. See more below.

VIDEO CAPSULE ENDOSCOPY

Okay, with EGD you can see the UGI tract and there is colonoscopy for the lower GI tract. The wireless video capsule endoscopy (VCE) is used to visualize the previously unvisualizable small bowel. It is especially useful in working up small bowel bleeds.

Typical scenario: patient presents with a history of episodic melanotic stools with negative EGDs and colonoscopies. Know!

The VCE is also finding more use in other small bowel problems such as assessing tumors, Crohn disease, and celiac disease.

BOWEL OBSTRUCTION

Obstruction: The most frequent cause of small intestine obstruction is post-operative adhesions. In decreasing order, the most common causes of colonic obstruction are: carcinoma, then diverticulitis, then volvulus.

The diagnosis of obstruction is made with a flat and upright abdominal film showing (typically) excessive amounts of air in the small bowel with no air in the colon. The presence of air fluid levels is helpful when there are "J-loops," in which the air fluid levels are at different heights on either side of the same loop of bowel. This signifies a dynamic obstruction. If the fluid levels are the same height on either side of the loop, paralytic ileus is the more likely diagnosis.

Treat with IV fluids and NG suction. Further workup is indicated if the symptoms do not resolve in 1–2 days. Gastrografin enema can be helpful if the obstruction is thought to be of colonic origin.

INTESTINAL ISCHEMIA

TYPES

There are 4 types of intestinal ischemia:
1) Colon ischemia (most common)
2) Chronic mesenteric ischemia
3) Acute mesenteric ischemia (70% mortality!)
4) Mesenteric venous thrombosis

COLON ISCHEMIA (ISCHEMIC COLITIS)

Colon ischemia (CI; ischemic colitis; colonic ischemia) is the most common form of intestinal ischemia. It is due to a non-occlusive ischemia—mostly involving some portions of the splenic flexure, descending colon, and/or sigmoid colon (i.e., inferior mesenteric circulation). Most often, no specific cause for the ischemia is found. It is a disease of the elderly and may be seen post-op (colonic surgery and aortic aneurysmectomy), and is occasionally associated with low-flow conditions (CHF) and hypercoagulable states. Because this condition is virtually never embolic, patients are not likely to have valvular heart disease or cardiac arrhythmia.

Symptoms of CI are usually a sudden LLQ pain with an urge to defecate, followed by passage of red-to-maroon stool within 1 day.

Mildest injury is mucosal and submucosal hemorrhage and edema—which is completely reversible. More severe injury ranges from replacement of mucosa and submucosa with granulation tissue to transmural infarction and fulminant colitis.

Submucosal hemorrhage and edema are seen on KUB or BE as "thumbprinting." This thumbprinting lasts only a few days and is not specific for the type of ischemia, just for submucosal edema or hem-orrhage.

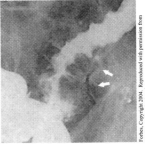

Image 1-26: Thumbprinting. Thickened mucosa is barely visible.

Forbes, Copyright 2004 - Reproduced with permission from Mosby, an Elsevier Imprint

Diagnose with colonoscopy if there are no signs of peritonitis. Also okay is sigmoidoscopy + gentle barium enema. Angi-ography is not done.

The usual treatment is bowel rest, fluids, and antibiotics. Most will resolve. Rare cases develop stricture or acute abdomen.

CHRONIC MESENTERIC ISCHEMIA

Chronic mesenteric ischemia is also called intestinal angina. These patients may have the classic triad:
1) abdominal pain after meals
2) abdominal bruit
3) weight loss (from tolerating only smaller meals)

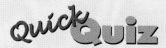

The pain is due to episodes of inadequate blood flow brought on by digestion.

Suspect mesenteric vascular ischemia in the above setting and especially if abdominal pain is out of proportion to any physical findings.

Symptoms are 1–3 hours of dull, gnawing abdominal pain beginning shortly after eating. The cause is atherosclerosis of the intestinal arteries with the symptoms caused by gastric "steal" after eating. Patients often have signs of other PVD and often have a smoking history.

Diagnosis is mainly based on symptoms. Many diagnostic tests have been tried, but none has proven very sensitive or specific. Even so, the workup includes MRA (magnetic resonance angiogram) or spiral CT. Splanchnic angiography is then done if these are abnormal.

Treatment is surgical bypass or angioplasty.

ACUTE MESENTERIC ISCHEMIA

Acute mesenteric ischemia (AMI) is the most severe form of intestinal ischemia with an average mortality rate of 70%—even with treatment! It results from acute loss of blood flow to part or all of the small intestine and/or ascending colon.

AMI is seen in older patients with a history of CHF, recent MI, cardiac arrhythmias, or hypotensive episodes.

Patients often have symptoms of intestinal angina (above) for months before the event. Because this condition is commonly embolic, patients are likely to have valvular heart disease or cardiac arrhythmia. These patients are acutely ill with vomiting, diarrhea, and occult blood.

Bowel infarction leads to acidosis, increased lactate, and elevated amylase. The abdominal exam may be fairly benign, leading to the erroneous diagnosis of acute gastroenteritis.

Do angiography unless there are signs of perforation (e.g., acidosis, high amylase)—in which case the patient goes directly to surgery for dead-bowel resection and possible embolectomy.

MESENTERIC VENOUS THROMBOSIS

Mesenteric venous thrombosis (MVT) is associated with hypercoagulable states, such as deficiencies of antithrombin III, prothrombin 20210 (a gene variant), protein S, and protein C and factor V Leiden defect.

MVT is also linked to
- pancreatitis
- intraabdominal sepsis
- paroxysmal nocturnal hemoglobinuria (PNH)
- liver disease (cirrhosis)
- sickle cell disease

MVT may be acute, subacute, or chronic. Like mesenteric infarction, the pain of MVT is often out of proportion to the abdominal exam. If the portal or splenic veins are involved in chronic MVT, there may be bleeding from gastroesophageal varices. CT is the diagnostic procedure of choice—with it > 90% of MVT can be diagnosed. Treat acute MVT with thrombolytics and long-term anticoagulants.

Treatment of chronic MVT is focused on minimizing bleeding from varices with sclerotherapy, portosystemic shunts, or similar devices.

CONSTIPATION

CAUSES

Causes of chronic constipation are many, but they usually result in:
- generalized or regional colonic inertia, and
- pelvic floor muscle dysfunction.

The large majority (> 90%) of cases are idiopathic! Lifestyle habits, such as a change to low-fiber diet; sudden, prolonged inactivity; and high stress may result in constipation.

Recent onset of constipation without change in lifestyle habits (e.g., no changes to diet, no new medications) suggests an obstructing lesion (neoplasm, stricture, foreign body). Pelvic floor dysfunction acts like outlet obstruction. Hysterectomy leads to refractory constipation in 5% of patients.

Neurologic causes affecting the parasympathetic innervation of the distal colon and rectum cause acquired megacolon; e.g., traumatic sacral nerve damage, MS, Chagas disease, or aganglionic megacolon (Hirschsprung). Chagas disease is found in Central and S. America. It is caused by infection with *Trypanosoma cruzi*, resulting in achalasia, cardiomyopathy, and acquired megacolon. Aganglionic megacolon (Hirschsprung) is usually diagnosed within the first 6 months of life, but a milder variant may present in adult patients.

Drugs with anticholinergic properties are common causes of constipation. These include antipsychotics, antidepressants, 1st generation antihistamines, and anticholinergic cold medications. Other causes include iron preparations, calcium supplements and calcium-channel blockers, and antacids containing aluminum or calcium.

Endocrine disorders, such as diabetes mellitus (DM) and hypothyroidism, often cause mild constipation. Myxedema may result in acquired megacolon. The altered progesterone and

notes

estrogen levels are the probable cause of constipation in **pregnancy**.

Collagen vascular diseases, especially progressive systemic sclerosis, are another cause of constipation.

Many of these causes can be revealed from a careful history.

DIAGNOSIS

Whom do you work up? Patients with constipation who additionally have weight loss, rectal bleeding, or anemia should get:

- Sigmoidoscopy + BE or a colonoscopy (to exclude structural disease; e.g., cancer, strictures)
- Serum Ca^{++} and TSH (to exclude hyper/hypocalcemia and hypothyroidism; DM is usually evident from the history).

For intractable constipation, test for colonic transit function. 20 radio-opaque markers ("Sitz markers") are taken by capsule, and a flat plate of the abdomen is done 5 days later. Normally, most markers are gone. It is abnormal for ≥ 5 to be retained. If the markers are spread throughout the colon, the cause is generalized colonic inertia. Clustering of markers in the rectosigmoid colon indicates pelvic floor dysfunction.

TREATMENT

Treatment consists of correcting any reversible cause. If idiopathic or irreversible, treatment is increasing dietary fiber to 25–30 gm/day and assuring fluid intake > 2.0 liters/day.

Note: Fiber or bulking agents often help with colonic inertia but **not** with pelvic floor dysfunction, which often responds to pelvic floor retraining (+/– biofeedback).

Increase exercise.

Short-term use of an osmotic laxative and/or stool softener is okay. Avoid stimulant laxatives.

Difficult cases usually respond well to daily use of polyethylene glycol powder with water or the recently approved lubiprostone (Amitiza®). Surgical treatment is indicated only for Hirschsprung disease.

FECAL IMPACTION

Fecal impaction is a large mass of dry, hard stool in the rectum causing constipation. Those at greatest risk are elderly with inadequate fluid intake who are also on narcotics or anticholinergics, or have decreased mobility.

Often, more proximal watery stool will leak around the impaction causing a watery fecal incontinence. Presentation is sudden onset of watery stools/incontinence in a person with chronic constipation.

Treatment is to remove the impaction. Initially, you can try a mineral oil enema, but often the impaction must be manually removed by breaking off small pieces until the obstruction is cleared. Longer-term treatment focuses on remedying the constipation: docusate stool softeners and bulk-forming agents used along with a bowel-training program (daily/regular BMs).

PANCREAS

ACUTE PANCREATITIS

Overview

Acute pancreatitis is usually caused by either alcohol abuse or gallstones, and it is believed these are the #1 and #2 etiologies in the U.S. In Europe, the reverse appears to be true as far as preponderant etiology. These are not firm conclusions; results from studies are influenced by where they are done. For example, if the study is done in a VA hospital, the primary cause will probably be alcohol abuse, whereas, if it is done in a community hospital, gallstones are more likely to cause the majority of cases.

Other causes of acute pancreatitis are acidosis (as in DKA), hypertriglyceridemia, hypercalcemia, trauma, and other problems that result in obstruction of the ampulla of Vater, such as pancreatic cancer.

Acute pancreatitis follows ERCP (see pg 1-1) in 5–20%.

Quite a few drugs can cause acute pancreatitis:

- diuretics: furosemide and the thiazides
- estrogens
- azathioprine
- antibiotics: tetracycline and the sulfonamides
- anti-HIV drugs, such as pentamidine and ddI
- oral hypoglycemics, 6-mercaptopurine, L-asparaginase, and valproic acid

Many initially "idiopathic" cases are due to biliary microlithiasis, cystic fibrosis, hereditary pancreatitis, or hypertriglyceridemia. Always check medications.

With acute pancreatitis, amylase and lipase are usually elevated. The serum amylase level is almost always elevated early on (> 3x N is almost always due to pancreatitis), but decreases within 2–3 days after disease onset. The lipase level increases later and stays elevated longer than the amylase at 7–14 days.

Very elevated serum or urine amylase levels, > 900 U/L and > 6000 U/L, respectively, are very specific indicators of acute pancreatitis (97%), but they have low sensitivity (50–70%).

High triglyceride level in the setting of acute pancreatitis may cause a spuriously normal amylase level! Additionally, triglyceride levels > 1000 mg/dL can cause pancreatitis.

Pancreatic Necrosis

The severity of acute pancreatitis is directly related to the degree of pancreatic necrosis (10% have necrosis) and whether this necrotic tissue is infected (mortality = 30%) or not (mortality = 10%). Overall, mortality rate for acute pancreatitis = 5–10%!

Severe pancreatitis causes multiple organ failure, which is reflected by:

- hemoconcentration,

notes

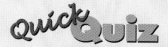
- heart: systolic BP < 90 mmHg; tachycardia > 130 bpm,
- lungs: PO_2 < 60 mmHg,
- renal: progressive azotemia or oliguria < 50 mL/hr,
- CNS = altered sensorium, and
- metabolic = low calcium (< 8 mg/dL) and albumin < 3.2 g/dL.

These indicators are used in several methods of assessment for severity that we will now discuss.

Assessing Severity

Okay, so we know severity of pancreatitis is associated with the degree of necrosis and signs of multiple organ failure. How do we determine severity on admission?

Three factors on admission are important indicators that the patient is more likely to have severe pancreatitis:

1) Overweight with a BMI > 25 (especially if obese with BMI of > 29).

2) Hemoconcentration with Hct > 50% in men and > 44% in women. This is one of the markers for multiple organ failure we just discussed. Follow serial Hct q 6 hours and if it is increasing or greater than these values, hydrate vigorously.

3) SIRS (systemic inflammatory response syndrome). This is basically a severe clinical response to an undefined insult (infectious or not) and not necessarily seen in multiple organ failure. SIRS is part of a somewhat newer method of categorizing severe illnesses. For instance, sepsis is defined as SIRS plus a documented or presumed infection. SIRS requires two or more of:

- temperature abnormal   (< 36°C or > 38°C)
- tachycardia   (HR > 90)
- tachypnea   (RR > 20 or pCO_2 < 32)
- WBC abnormal   (> 12,000/μL or < 4,000/μL or > 10% bands)

Signs of organ failure are also used in the APACHE II and III systems. The APACHE scores are more sensitive and specific than the previous methods used but require a computer to figure and are not embraced by many. They are used in ICUs.

Skin findings:

The most common skin finding is an erythema of the flanks caused by extravasated pancreatic exudates.

Cullen sign and Turner sign, when seen (unusual), indicate a severe necrotizing pancreatitis.

- Cullen sign, a faint blue discoloration around the umbilicus, indicates hemoperitoneum, while
- Turner (or Grey-Turner) sign, a bluish-reddish-purple or greenish-brown discoloration of the flanks, results from tissue catabolism of hemoglobin from retroperitoneal blood dissecting along the tissue planes.

These are characteristic but not pathognomonic of acute pancreatitis. Cullen sign is also seen with intraperitoneal bleeding (esp. ruptured ectopic pregnancy), and Turner sign is seen with other causes of retroperitoneal bleeding.

Pancreatic necrosis is best confirmed by dynamic CT scan or MRI (at some centers). It is considered severe if ≥ 30% of the pancreas is necrotic.

When following after admission, you simply do a SIRS evaluation daily and look for signs of multiple organ failure. Worsening indicators indicate worsening severity. ICUs may also use the APACHE system.

Fluid / Masses in Acute Pancreatitis

[Know!]

- Acute fluid collections with high amylase levels appear in up to 50% of patients within 48 hours of pain onset. They usually resolve spontaneously. A sympathetic transudative left pleural effusion frequently occurs. Rarely, a diaphragmatic defect into the pleural space causes an effusion high in amylase. (See Figure 1-4)

- Inflamed, edematous, necrotic pancreas occurs in the first 1-2 weeks, and may simulate a pseudocyst (which usually occurs later; discussed below). It can additionally be differ-entiated from a pseudocyst by ultrasonography. This condition is serious and may require drainage.

- Infected pancreatic necrosis usually requires surgery within 2 weeks of the episode. You can diagnose by CT-guided aspiration of necrotic pancreas with bacterial smear and culture.

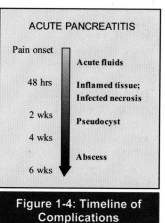

ACUTE PANCREATITIS

Pain onset	
	Acute fluids
48 hrs	Inflamed tissue; Infected necrosis
2 wks	Pseudocyst
4 wks	
	Abscess
6 wks	

Figure 1-4: Timeline of Complications

notes

- A pancreatic **pseudocyst** develops in 10–15% of patients with acute pancreatitis. It requires 2–4 weeks to develop after the acute attack. Basically, it is a collection of pancreatic fluid which, if small enough, resolves spontaneously. A size > 5 cm suggests it may not resolve. If the pseudocyst persists > 3–6 months, it will probably require surgical drainage.

  Remove **enlarging** pseudocysts because they are associated with serious complications—especially fistula, pseudoaneurysms, rupture, and hemorrhage. Rupture without hemorrhage = 15% mortality, while rupture with hemorrhage = 60% mortality! Consider this in a patient who is recovering normally and then suddenly gets worse.

- A pancreatic **abscess** occurs 4–6 weeks after onset of acute severe pancreatitis—in which there is severe pancreatic necrosis. It may be seen as a "soap bubble sign" on upright abdominal x-ray. This is a very serious condition with fever and shock.

  Diagnose pancreatic abscess with Gram stain of a CT-directed percutaneous aspiration—which is 90% accurate. This allows for immediate surgical debridement and drainage.

Diagnosis

In working up the **cause** of acute pancreatitis, the first test and often only test is gallbladder ultrasound to rule out gallstones. Diagnosis is often based mainly on history.

Treatment of Acute Pancreatitis

Treatment: ~ 90% resolve spontaneously within a few days with supportive care. Patients must be made NPO, but NG **suction** is generally **not** required. IV fluids and colloids, as needed. **Enteral feeds** have been shown to be **superior to TPN** in maintaining nutritional status in patients with protracted acute pancreatitis.

Give systemic antibiotics if there is established infection or severe pancreatitis with any organ failure or ≥ 30% pancreatic necrosis. Use antibiotics that are excreted in the pancreas; e.g., imipenem or cefuroxime.

Be wary of antibiotic-associated fungal infections.

Pearls of Acute Pancreatitis

Acute pancreatitis pearls:
- If the amylase is still elevated after 10 days, think of something else going on, such as a leaking pseudocyst. With large fluid collections, consider a disrupted pancre-atic duct leaking fluid. This can be treated by ERCP with stenting of the duct.
- Recurrent acute pancreatitis with no evidence of gallstones or alcohol abuse may be due to **microlithiasis**; thus, consider an elective cholecystectomy.
- Gastric varices in the absence of esophageal varices occur only in **splenic vein thrombosis**, which is a complication of both severe **acute** pancreatitis and **chronic** pancreatitis.

- ERCP is not done acutely unless a patient has cholangitis and sepsis. Use ERCP after the acute period to exclude or treat any suspected common duct stones (e.g., the bilirubin is > 2.5 and rising or the ultrasound shows a dilated common duct). Perform cholecystectomy ASAP after gallstone pancreatitis—after the inflammation has resolved.

- Criteria for resumption of oral feeds in acute pancreatitis:
  - bowel sounds present and passing flatus/stools
  - not requiring narcotics
  - patient expresses hunger

Question: What conditions can cause abdominal pain with an elevated amylase? Answer: Acute pancreatitis, acute cholecystitis, intestinal infarction, diabetic ketoacidosis, perforated ulcer, salpingitis, and ectopic pregnancy! Other causes of hyperamylasemia are increased salivary amylase and macroamylasemia (a benign condition due to a low urinary excretion of amylase).

CHRONIC PANCREATITIS

Overview

Chronic pancreatitis is, in developed countries, usually (60–70%) a result of chronic alcohol ingestion—typically > 10 years. Next in frequency is idiopathic (30%), and about 10% are rare hereditary disorders (lack of cationic trypsinogen activator inhibitor, SPINK abnormality) and other causes such as cystic fibrosis, pancreas divisum, tumor, and hyperparathyroidism. Autoimmune pancreatitis (described below) is a newly described rare disorder that accounts for less than 1% of cases.

There is an initial, asymptomatic phase, followed by recurrent bouts of abdominal pain. Late in the disease, when > 80–90% of the endocrine and exocrine function is lost, patients develop steatorrhea and diabetes. The fecal fat in these late-stage patients is higher than with other disorders—it may be > 100 gm/day. > 40 gm/day is highly suggestive of chronic pancreatitis. 1/3 of patients with chronic pancreatitis develop diabetes (see below). Chronic pancreatitis also increases the risk of pancreatic cancer two-fold—not high enough to do screening exams.

Diagnosis

The classic diagnostic triad for chronic pancreatitis is:
1) pancreatic calcification,
2) diabetes, and
3) steatorrhea.

Diagnosis can be difficult, so begin evaluation with simple, noninvasive tests that detect advanced forms of chronic pancreatitis. First, get a CT of the abdomen and a serum trypsin level—if the pancreas is calcified, or if the serum trypsin is abnormally low, you have made the diagnosis of chronic pancreatitis!

notes

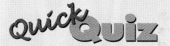
Key tests used in the diagnosis of chronic pancreatitis are:
- abdominal CT has an 80%/85% sensitivity and specificity and is the current procedure of choice;
- endoscopic ultrasound (EUS)—very sensitive and may be the best test yet. But it requires a very skilled gastroenterologist. It is the procedure of choice in some centers;
- abdominal U/S;
- flat plate of the abdomen showing pancreatic calcification has only 30% sensitivity; and
- secretin stimulation test (see below).

2nd level. If results from the tests above are negative, and you still have suspicions, do either magnetic resonance cholangiopancreatography (MRCP; preferred) or ERCP:
- MRCP is accurate in diagnosing chronic pancreatitis without the risk of inducing pancreatitis (5–20%), as with ERCP. MRCP additionally visualizes the biliary tree and thus can also be useful in some cases of suspected bile duct stones or other biliary diseases like PSC. MRCP is the preferred 2nd level test.
- ERCP is likely to induce pancreatitis. The only advantage ERCP has is when there are calcific stones present within the duct that are amenable to endoscopic removal.

Both show large duct disease **and** small duct disease. With large duct disease, the pancreatic duct has stenoses and dilations, which visualize as an irregular "chain of lakes."

Dilation of the common bile duct can be caused by chronic pancreatitis but also by pancreatic cancer. Either can compress the downstream portion of the common bile duct as it passes through the head of the pancreas.

The secretin test is the most sensitive test for pancreatic function; however, it is complicated, so it is usually performed only in major medical centers, and only when there is still a high "index of suspicion" after negative 2nd level tests (this does vary—in some places with ready access, it is done before ERCP). In this test, IV infusion of secretin (+/- cholecystokinin [CCK]) causes a direct stimulation of the pancreas. Duodenal pancreatic secretions are then measured via a tube. The bicarbonate concentration should be > 80 mEq/L. CCK stimulates lipase, amylase, trypsin, and chymotrypsin, which can also be measured. An endoscopic secretin test is now available.

Several breath tests for assessing pancreatic function are undergoing evaluation. 2 of these are the cholesteryl-[14C] octanoate breath test and the HPLCN-benzoyl-tyrosyl-p-aminobenzoic acid/p-aminosalicylic acid (NBT-PABA/PAS) test. The results are promising, and they may replace more invasive tests in the future.

Complications of Chronic Pancreatitis

A major complication is persistent and severe abdominal pain. In this setting:
- rule out continued ETOH use;
- rule out pseudocyst;
- do an MRCP, EUS, or ERCP (least preferred) to define duct anatomy; and
- try high-dose pancreatic enzymes to shut off the enteropancreatic (intestine-pancreas) axis.

Pancreatic cancer develops in 4% of patients with chronic pancreatitis > 20 years.

Complications of chronic pancreatitis include gastric varices (from splenic vein thrombosis), B_{12} malabsorption, jaundice, pleural effusion, and brittle diabetes mellitus. The only skin involvement is tender red nodules from fat necrosis; this is uncommon, but can simulate erythema nodosum.

The diabetes associated with chronic pancreatitis is different from the usual DM. It occurs when > 80% of the pancreas is destroyed. There is a decrease in production of insulin and glucagon.

Because the pancreas is producing so little glucagon, the patient is very prone to hypoglycemia. Therefore, less stringent control of hyperglycemia is recommended—to decrease the chance of a hypoglycemic episode.

These patients do not have the retinopathy and nephropathy associated with the usual DM. They commonly have neuropathy, but it is more likely caused by alcoholism and/or malnutrition.

Treatment of Chronic Pancreatitis

Treatment includes pancreatic enzymes (20,000–30,000 units of lipase/day), decreasing dietary fat, and adding medium-chain triglycerides to the diet. Pancreatic enzymes must either have an enteric coating or be given with antacids/H_2 blockers because gastric acid destroys enzymes.

Analgesia is sometimes required. Usually a short-term opioid with amitriptyline is tried. There is no therapy proven to show benefit if the pain continues.

notes

AUTOIMMUNE PANCREATITIS

This is a newly described entity that you should know about even though it occurs in < 1% of cases of chronic pancreatitis. It is interesting in that its presentation often simulates cancer of the pancreas. What to know:

- 70% present with obstructive jaundice (simulating cancer of the pancreas).
- CT can show a mass in the head of the pancreas (again simulating cancer) or diffuse enlargement.
- There may be bile duct and pancreatic duct strictures.
- Serum IgG4 level is specific and usually markedly elevated.

Histology shows a dense lymphoplasmacytic infiltrate. Treatment is corticosteroids.

PANCREATIC NEOPLASMS

Pancreatic Cancer

Pancreatic cancer is astonishingly aggressive. 80% of patients present with advanced disease. Heavy smokers have 2x N risk. Other risk factors include DM, pancreatic cancer in 2 first-order relatives, hereditary pancreatitis, and chronic pancreatitis.

Patients usually present with some combination of jaundice, unexplained upper abdominal pain, and/or weight loss.

Where the cancer is located affects presenting signs and stage:

- Head: Painless jaundice tends to be the presenting sign with early-stage cancers of the head of the pancreas.
- Body and tail: These patients are more likely to present with pain and weight loss (jaundice in only ~ 30%) and with the cancer at a much more advanced stage.

Pain and weight loss are indications of advanced disease. The pain typically has a gnawing quality, is not cured by eating, and occasionally radiates to the back.

Diagnosis is made using helical CT, CT angiography, endoscopic ultrasound (EUS)-guided FNA biopsy, and laparoscopy. Note: There is some controversy concerning FNA biopsy possibly seeding the tumor.

The most used and very accurate serum marker is the concentration of cancer-associated antigen 19-9 (CA 19-9).

Most common reasons for being unresectable:

- distant metastases
- local invasion of major vessel (portal vessel or superior mesenteric vein or artery)

Treatment of pancreatic cancer: Resection is the only hope for cure.

Basically, if the patient is a surgical candidate, has a mass in the head of the pancreas, and the cancer appears resectable, a pancreaticoduodenectomy (Whipple resection) is done, and lymph nodes are checked at the time of surgery—at which time you find out if they are node-negative or node-positive.

There is (as yet) no clear survival benefit, but adjuvant chemo-radiotherapy (especially with 5-FU or gemcitabine) is usually offered.

If non-invasive workup shows that the cancer has already metastasized, avoid surgery—do supportive care or give experimental chemo (especially gemcitabine) only. Put a stent in with ERCP for biliary obstruction. This is the only time you use ERCP for pancreatic cancer.

Post-surgical prognosis: 5-year survival is 30% for node-negative; 10% for node-positive.

Glucagonoma

A glucagonoma is a glucagon-secreting, alpha-cell tumor of the pancreas that causes a unique set of clinical findings. These are very distinctive: scaly necrolytic erythema, weight loss, anemia, and persistent hyperglycemia. Plasma glucagon (by RIA) is usually > 1000 pg/dL.

Insulinoma

Insulinoma is a very rare, insulin-secreting beta-cell tumor of the pancreas. This is covered in the Endocrinology section (under Hypoglycemia).

Gastrinoma

Gastrinomas are discussed under ZE syndrome on pg 1-13. Most (50%) are found in the duodenum, 24% in the pancreas. This diagnosis is likely when the serum gastrin is > 500 and gastric acid is present.

VIPoma

VIPomas: Tumors that secrete vasoactive intestinal peptide (VIP). 2/3 occur in the pancreas, and > 1/2 of them are malignant. They cause a profuse secretory diarrhea ("pancreatic cholera"). Diagnosis: increased serum VIP level and hypokalemia.

BILIARY SYSTEM

CHOLELITHIASIS

Overview

Cholelithiasis is widespread—20% of women and 8% of men—and usually asymptomatic. It is not associated with hypercholesterolemia.

The pathophysiology of cholelithiasis involves 1 or more of the following 3 factors:

1) abnormal (lithogenic—supersaturated with cholesterol) bile secreted by the liver
2) accelerated nucleation of microcrystals to macrocrystals
3) defective gall bladder emptying

Cholelithiasis has been associated with obesity, oral contraceptive use, clofibrate treatment, and ileal disease or resection. 80% of gallstones are composed of radiolucent cholesterol, and the remainder are of pigment.

notes

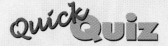
Profile for cholesterol stones: Rapid weight loss in obese patient (these stones prevented by aspirin or ursodeoxycholic acid), American Indian, octreotide use.

Profile for pigment stones: Ileal resection (as in Crohn disease), sickle cell disease, or anything else that causes hemolysis (e.g. *Clonorchis* biliary dwelling trematode).

Symptoms: RUQ pain lasting 20–60 minutes—especially after a fatty meal. But fatty food intolerance is a very nonspecific finding

Diagnosis of Cholelithiasis

To detect the presence of stones, do an ultrasound (90% sensitive). A normal ultrasound in the presence of normal bilirubin and liver enzymes is sensitive for excluding common duct stones. If the ultrasound is technically inadequate, consider MRCP or oral cholecystogram. The usual procedures used for diagnosing common duct obstruction are MRCP, ERCP, and transhepatic cholangiography.

The HIDA scan (cholescintigraphy) is the best test for confirming acute cystic duct obstruction (i.e., acute cholecystitis) by imaging of the bile duct but not the gallbladder, although ultrasound has characteristic findings of acute cholecystitis.

Note: About half of pigment stones are radio-opaque, whereas cholesterol stones never are.

Treatment of Cholelithiasis

If the patient has gallstones and is symptomatic, do an elective cholecystectomy because 70% of these patients have recurrent symptoms if not treated.

If a patient has gallbladder stones but is asymptomatic, no treatment is indicated because only 20% subsequently develop symptoms within 10–20 years. Don't mistake symptoms of reflux for that of cholelithiasis, even if you incidentally find stones in the gallbladder.

Supplemental oral bile acid (ursodeoxycholic acid) is "successful" in the treatment of cholesterol stones only; and only if the stones are < 1 cm, radiolucent, few in number, and the patient is compliant. Even so, the stones usually recur anyway! Not used much. There is no real role for lithotripsy.

Acalculous cholecystitis occurs only in seriously ill patients (e.g., major trauma, burns, after major surgeries). Diagnosis may be assisted by ultrasound or CT showing no stones, but a large, tense, often thickened gallbladder with pericholecystic fluid (or no stones and a HIDA scan showing cystic duct obstruction). Treatment is cholecystectomy but cholecystostomy can be done if the patient is too sick for surgery.

Common Duct Stones

Alk phos and bilirubin levels usually do not increase in typical gallbladder cases because the gallstones block only the exit to the gallbladder. Increasing levels of alk phos and bili suggest a common duct stone. Consider common duct stone in the gallbladder patient with increased alk phos and bili or the post-cholecystectomy patient with persistent pain.

Common duct stones are removed by ERCP with prn endoscopic sphincterotomy.

CHOLESTASIS

Cholestasis can be obstructive (as with common duct stones) or hepatocellular. In both cases, there is retention of the substances normally released into bile. In both cases, there are "cholestatic" LFTs with increased alkaline phosphatase and conjugated bilirubin with bilirubinuria. More on bilirubin on pg 1-52.

CHOLANGITIS

Cholangitis is a complication of common bile duct blockage. Acute cholangitis is suggested by the triad of biliary colic, fever and chills, and jaundice (Charcot's triad). Suppurative cholangitis additionally has mental confusion, bacteremia, and septic shock. Antibiotics are indicated but are not sufficient treatment for suppurative cholangitis. When you suspect suppurative cholangitis, the best procedure for both diagnosis and treatment is ERCP with endoscopic sphincterotomy or surgery if ERCP is not available.

Emphysematous cholecystitis requires emergent laparotomy with cholecystectomy and antibiotics. In both suppurative cases, the antibiotics must be effective against both Gram-negative and anaerobic organisms. Do not use ceftriaxone—it can cause biliary concrements!

PORCELAIN GALLBLADDER

X-ray showing a gallbladder with a calcified outline ("porcelain gallbladder") suggests cancer, and an open cholecystectomy is indicated.

PRIMARY BILIARY CIRRHOSIS

Overview

Primary Biliary Cirrhosis (PBC): Slow onset. Usually occurs in middle-aged women. PBC is characterized by a non-suppurative, progressive, destructive cholangiolitis. The cause of PBC is unknown, but 70% have associated diseases of altered immunity (e.g., Sjögren's, scleroderma, autoimmune thyroiditis, limited scleroderma), and the disease does

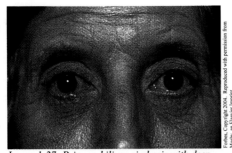

Image 1-27: Primary biliary cirrhosis with deep jaundice, brown pigmentation, spider nevi, and xanthelasmata.

run in families. 90% have a positive antimitochondrial antibody test (> 1:40), but degree of elevation does not correlate with severity of disease.

The bile ducts become chronically inflamed and eventually cause obstructive jaundice and liver cirrhosis.

Symptoms: Patients who present with symptoms have advanced disease. The majority of patients present asymptomatically and are worked up because of a high alkaline phosphatase noted on a liver function screening. If they have symptoms, patients initially complain of itching—first in the palms and soles and later throughout the body. They later develop jaundice, hyperpigmentation, vitamin D-dependent osteomalacia, and accelerated osteoporosis.

They can get xanthomas and xanthelasmas from the hypercholesterolemia (but this does not convey increased risk of CAD because there is also an elevated HDL).

The disease is indolent, but relentlessly progressive. Symptomatic patients have a median survival of 10 years, and asymptomatic patients live much longer. When the bilirubin is > 2, the disease accelerates. Most die soon after the bilirubin reaches 10 unless the patient undergoes liver transplantation.

Incidental discovery of a 2–5x increase in serum alkaline phosphatase has been the main stimulus for the increase in PBC diagnoses. High levels of alk phos occur in up to 95% of patients with PBC.

Note: The antimitochondrial antibody test is the hallmark test for PBC. Even so, it is not a good indicator of the severity of PBC. The antimitochondrial antibody test is only occasionally positive in both autoimmune hepatitis and drug-induced chronic hepatitis; a high titer in a patient with autoimmune hepatitis suggests an overlap syndrome. (See Table 1-8)

Table 1-8: Serologic Markers in PBC and CAH			
	Primary Biliary Cirrhosis	Drug-induced CAH	Autoimmune CAH
Antimitochondrial Ab	90-95% Positive	occ Positive	occ Positive (low titers)
Anti-Smooth muscle Ab	Negative	Negative	Positive
Antinuclear Ab	usu Negative	Negative	Positive

Diagnosis of Biliary Cirrhosis

Diagnosis is confirmed only with a liver biopsy, which may show granulomas (often it has nonspecific findings). PBC patients also have a high hepatic copper level (but so do those with primary sclerosing cholangitis and Wilson disease).

Treatment of Biliary Cirrhosis

Ursodiol (ursodeoxycholate—a synthetic bile acid) is the best proven treatment available for PBC. It improves LFTs and decreases symptoms, and it may delay (but not prevent) progression of the disease. Otherwise, there is just symptomatic treatment. For pruritus: cholestyramine. For osteomalacia: Vitamin D, estrogen, and calcium. For malabsorption: medium-chain triglycerides and decreased dietary fat. Treatment has no effect on late disease.

For late disease, liver transplantation is the recommended procedure. It has been shown to significantly improve survival in late PBC. PBC is one of the most common disease indications for liver transplantation (hepatitis C is the most common)! The "AAAABCs of PBC" are: Antimitochondrial Antibody Attack increases Alk phos and causes Biliary lesions and Cirrhosis.

PRIMARY SCLEROSING CHOLANGITIS

Overview

Primary Sclerosing Cholangitis (PSC): Also indolent. It primarily occurs in males (70%) with average age of 45. It has a strong association with colitis (75%!)—so it is mainly seen in ulcerative colitis but can occur in Crohn disease involving the colon. It has no relation to the severity of colitis.

UC may precede the diagnosis of PSC, and all PSC patients should have a colonoscopy. Conversely, PSC may precede the diagnosis of UC; therefore all UC patients who have a persistent ≥ 2x increase in alkaline phosphatase should be screened for PSC.

Cause is unknown. Patients develop inflammation and sclerosis of the entire biliary tract (intra- and extrahepatic), leading to obstructive jaundice and eventually cirrhosis. Bilirubin and alkaline phosphatase levels are elevated (cholestatic pattern). There is an elevated hepatic copper level (as in primary biliary cirrhosis and Wilson disease), but the antimitochondrial antibody is negative. The total protein level gives an idea of how much the disease has affected liver function.

Patients are initially asymptomatic but eventually, with advanced disease, develop weakness and fatigue, abdominal pain, itching, and jaundice.

8–15% of PSC patients develop cholangiocarcinoma. One third have it when first diagnosed with PSC! Suspect if symptoms of PSC abruptly worsen. CA 19-9 is elevated in 80%.

Diagnosis of Sclerosing Cholangitis

Diagnosis of PSC is made with MRCP (best), ERCP, or transhepatic cholangiography. These reveal irregularly narrowed bile ducts with small bile duct ballooning just prior to ob-

notes

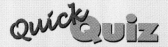

Quick Quiz

1) What is the "hallmark" test for primary biliary cirrhosis? How do you confirm the diagnosis?

2) PBC: What is the best, proven treatment for early disease? For late disease?

3) List the similarities and differences between PBC and PSC. Commonly confused diseases. [Know!] What are the alk phos, bilirubin, hepatic copper, and antimitochondrial antibody tests in PBC and PSC?

4) A patient presents with cholestatic jaundice and a history of IBD (or a history of chronic diarrhea). Which of the following do you include in your differential— PBC or PSC? Why?

structions, producing the typical "beaded" appearance. With ERCP, if a dominant stricture exists, it can be dilated. Liver biopsy will show "onion skin" fibrosis in portal triads.

In small duct PSC, the extrahepatic and intrahepatic biliary system may be nondiagnostic, but liver biopsy abnormalities establish the diagnosis.

Secondary causes of sclerosing cholangitis must be ruled out. These include: bacterial cholangitis (stones or bile duct stricture), atypical anatomy (congenital or previous surgery), bile duct neoplasms, and AIDS-associated cholangiopathy.

Treatment of Sclerosing Cholangitis

Treatment of PSC: The only sure treatment for PSC is a liver transplant; although colectomy cures ulcerative colitis, it does not change the course of this associated disease. High-dose ursodeoxycholic acid (20–25 mg/kg) may retard progression of disease.

Remember: When a patient presents with jaundice and increased alk phos and has history of chronic diarrhea or IBD, especially UC, rule out PSC with ERCP!

Again: PSC: Sclerosing Cholangitis, colitis, cholestatic bili and alk phos levels, and endoscopic retrograde cholangiopancreatography (ERCP).

PBC VS. PSC

These two conditions are often confused. To help remember, drop the abbreviations and think:

Both have jaundice and high alkaline phosphatase.

Biliary cirrhosis: 55-year-old woman named Hillary C. Roses with fatigue and pruritus. Antimitochondrial Ab +.

Sclerosing cholangitis: 45-year-old man with UC.

PBC middle aged women

LIVER

HEPATITIS NOTES

Hepatitis: ALT (SGPT) is more liver-specific than AST (SGOT). To remember that ALT is the more liver-specific, think of "L-L": "ALT-Liver."
- With alcoholic hepatitis, the AST:ALT is about 3:1 because the alcohol damages mitochondria, which are a source of AST, and is less liver-specific.
- With viral hepatitis, the ALT is usually greater than the AST because its toxicity is more liver-specific. Table 1-10 reviews the hepatitis serological tests.
- Nonalcoholic fatty liver disease (NAFLD) is also more liver-specific and has an ALT:AST ratio > 2:1.

Acute viral hepatitis has histologic characteristics of diffuse liver cell injury and swelling, increased macrophages, accelerated apoptosis (the normal programmed cell death is accelerated by viral hepatitis), and inflammatory periportal infiltrates (mostly lymphocytic).

Chronic viral hepatitis has histologic characteristics of interface hepatitis (formerly known as piecemeal necrosis) and fibrosis.

EVALUATION OF ABNORMAL LIVER BIOCHEMICAL TESTS

Increased Transaminases

An abnormal laboratory value should be confirmed before ordering specific tests. If confirmed, order a full set of liver biochemical tests, including alkaline phosphatase, total and direct bilirubin, albumin, PT, and CBC. If at this time the transaminases are still elevated, order more specific tests for hepatitis A, B, and C—and tests for hemochromatosis to include iron studies and ferritin level.

Increased Alkaline Phosphatase

Remember that alkaline phosphatase comes from liver and bones. Gamma glutamyl transpeptidase (GGT) usually rises in parallel with alkaline phosphatase from the liver and should be checked in cases of increased alkaline phosphatase with normal bilirubin and transaminases. Generally, the next test is abdominal ultrasound to look for dilated biliary ducts or metastatic liver lesions. In appropriate patients, also order anti-mitochondrial antibody test (to screen for PBC).

HEPATITIS B

Overview

[Know]: The 5 main serological markers in hepatitis B are HBsAg, HBsAb, HBcAb, HBeAg, and HBeAb. See Table 1-9 and Table 1-10.
- HBsAg: There are 3 HBsAg+ proteins seen in the serum in patients with hepatitis B: one large, double-shelled 42 nm particle that is the intact virion and two smaller 22 nm

notes

spherical or rod-shaped protein particles that outnumber the large particle by up to 1000 to 1! These 22 nm HBsAg+ particles are thought to be just excess viral coat protein. The HBsAg has many different subtypes (adw, adr) that have no clinical significance, although they are used epidemiologically to evaluate outbreaks. Finding HBsAb in the serum indicates past exposure to either hepatitis B virion or to the vaccine.

• HBcAg+ protein is the core particle (inner shell) of the above 42 nm virion. This protein is retained in the hepatocyte until it is covered with HBsAg+ nucleocapsid outer shell, which will then incorporate the DNA. Free HBcAg+ protein does not circulate in the serum. Antibody to HBcAg appears early in the disease (initially IgM, then IgG) and persists for life, so HBcAb IgG is the best marker for previous exposure to HBV.

• HBeAg is a soluble protein made from the same gene as HBcAg but, unlike HBcAg, HBeAg is secreted from the hepatocytes and circulated in the serum. It correlates with the quantity of intact virus and, therefore, with infectivity and liver inflammation. The HBe antibody (HBeAb) appears several weeks after the illness. Detecting HBsAg and HBeAg indicates active virions and high infectivity (more so than HBsAg+ and HBeAg-). The tests for HBeAg and HBeAb are often not available locally.

Hepatitis B is the only hepatitis virus composed of DNA. Incubation period is 1–6 months. It is transmitted by contaminated serum or blood products. Once infected, the first marker detectable in the serum is the antigen HBsAg. This is followed by the appearance of antibody to the core antigen. After HBsAg becomes undetectable, there is a period of weeks to months before the HBsAb antibody becomes detectable. This is called the "window," and you must perform an HBcAb IgM test during this period to confirm acute hepatitis B. See Figure 1-5 and Table 1-9.

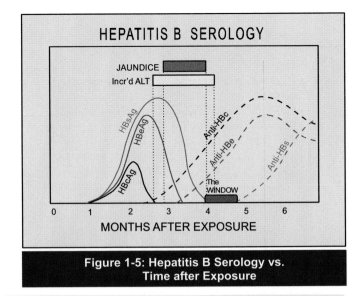

Figure 1-5: Hepatitis B Serology vs. Time after Exposure

Hepatitis B is strongly associated with polyarteritis nodosa (PAN). The surface antigen is found in 20–30% of these patients. It appears that the hepatitis B infection precipitates an autoimmune reaction resulting in PAN.

Clinical: First, there are prodromal constitutional symptoms, which typically resolve at the time jaundice becomes apparent. Occasionally (10–15%), the prodromal symptoms are serum sickness-like with fever, arthritis, urticaria, and angioedema. This seems to be caused by circulating immune complexes (especially "HBsAg—HBsAb" immune complex) activating the complement system. With the onset of jaundice, the patient usually feels much better, but may have liver swelling and tenderness and cholestatic symptoms.

Removal of HBV is T-cell-mediated, and the only purpose of HBsAb is to prevent reinfection.

Hepatitis B immune globulin (HBIG; HBsAb) provides some protection against hepatitis B, although it appears to only de-

HBsAg	Anti-HBc	Anti-HBs	Interpretation
+	–	–	Acute Infection
+	+	–	3 poss: 1) Acute infection 2) Chronic Hep B (high AST) 3) Inactive carrier (normal enzymes)
–	–	+	2 poss: 1) Remote infection 2) Immunized
–	+	+	Remote infection
–	+	–	3 poss: 1) Window disease 2) Remote infection 3) False positive
+	+	+	More than 1 infection. E.g., IV drug user or renal dialysis patient with both acute and chronic hepatitis B (infected with different strains of hepatitis B).

Table 1-9: Interpretation of Hepatitis B Tests

notes

crease the severity of illness rather than protect the patient from disease.

HBIG is effective both as prophylaxis and when given in early infection.

Hepatitis B Vaccines

The 2 hepatitis B vaccines are composed of HBsAg. They are equally effective and are safe for pregnant patients. It is best if the hepatitis B vaccine is given before the patient is exposed to HBV. 95% of immunocompetent patients develop antibodies, whereas only about 50% of dialysis patients do. Because these vaccines are surface antigens, to ensure effectiveness after the course of vaccine has been given, check for HBsAb—there will be no HBcAb.

Chronic Hepatitis B

The likelihood of developing chronic HBV is inversely related to age. Chronic HBV occurs in 90% of infants infected at birth, 25–50% in children age 1–5 years, and 5% in older children and adults.

There is now universal preschool vaccination in the U.S. Overall, < 1% of patients with hepatitis B develop fulminant hepatitis, but 5–7% develop chronic carrier states.

There are 2 types of hepatitis B carrier states:
1) inactive carrier state (asymptomatic with normal liver enzymes)
2) chronic hepatitis B (abnormal enzymes)

A liver biopsy is usually required to confirm the diagnosis of chronic hepatitis B.

Patients with inactive carrier states can develop severe exacerbations of hepatitis B if they become immunocompromised. For example, a woman with breast cancer who also has an inactive carrier state with hepatitis B is to be started on chemotherapy. What other drug is given? Lamivudine is given with her chemotherapy to blunt viral replication.

Chronic hepatitis B is a serious illness—it often progresses to cirrhosis and is strongly associated with hepatocellular cancer (HCC). Lifetime risk for HCC is 20% so screen q 6 mo with alpha-fetoprotein and ultrasound (just as we do with chronic hepatitis C and alcoholic liver disease).

Hepatitis B Treatment Scenarios

Scenarios:
- Give a newborn of a mother with hepatitis B, hepatitis B immune globulin (HBIG) and hepatitis B vaccination. There is a 5–10% transplacental transmission of HBV.
- If an asymptomatic patient has HBsAg in the serum, it means either the patient is a carrier or the patient has early hepatitis B—so initial action is only to follow closely (once the patient is infected, neither vaccine nor HBIG helps).
- Close contacts of a patient with acute HBV infection should be given HBIG followed by a complete course of HBV vaccinations. This includes sexual contacts and household contacts of the patient. Pregnant women are treated the same.

	HAVAb IgM	HAVAb IgG	HBsAg	HBsAb IgG	HBcAb IgG	HBcAb IgM	HBeAg	HDVAb
Table 1-10: Hepatitis—Serological Tests								
Acute Hepatitis A	+	−			−			
Previous HAV	−	+			−			
Acute HBV			+ early	−	−	+	+	−
Acute HBV − window			−	−	−	+	−	−
Chronic active HBV			+	−	+	−	usu +	−
Remote HBV (immune)			−	+	+	−	−	−
Vaccinated (immune)	−		−	+	−	−	−	−
Acute Hepatitis D (w acute HB)			+ early	−	−	+	+	+
Acute Hepatitis D (w CAH)			+	rarely	+	−	usu +	+

Table 1-11: Treatment of Chronic Active Hepatitis B			
Treatment	**Benefits**	**Disadvantages**	**Used for**
Interferon	Limited duration of therapy. 35% complete remission. No resistance. Potent.	Side effects may be severe. Contraindicated in decompensated liver disease.	Primary treatment for young patients and women contemplating pregnancy
Entecavir	Low drug resistance	Potent antiviral	Primary treatment
Lamivudine	Great safety profile, even in pregnancy	High rate of drug resistance	Primary treatment
Adefovir	Active against lamivudine-resistant HBV	Low viral suppression	Lamivudine-resistant HBV
Telbivudine	Slightly more potent than adefovir and entecavir	Same resistance profile as lamivudine	Not used much

Note: Several months after an episode of hepatitis B infection, check for loss of HBsAg and HBV-DNA to ensure that it has not become a chronic infection.

Treatment of Chronic Active Hepatitis B

Who Should Be Treated

HBV DNA, ALT, HBeAg, and degree of cirrhosis are used to determine when to treat. Treatment is recommended for:
All those with HBV DNA > 20,000 and ALT > 2 x ULN
• Treatment is started immediately for HBeAg– .
• Treatment is delayed 3–6 months for newly diagnosed HBeAg+ patients to see if seroconversion takes place.

The presence of cirrhosis requires less HBV DNA to initiate treatment. Treat:
• Compensated cirrhosis and HBV DNA > 2000
• Decompensated cirrhosis and detectable HBV DNA

See Table 1-11 for treatment options for CAH B.
Liver transplantation is the only treatment for end-stage liver disease. The HBV recurs in the transplanted liver, but an anti-viral treatment program can help.

HEPATITIS A

Hepatitis A is an RNA virus. It is easily transmitted fecal-orally—usually via food or water. It can be sexually transmitted. There is no transplacental transmission! There are no carrier or persistent states although, occasionally, these patients get prolonged cholestasis (with increased bili and alk phos) for up to 4 months. Incubation period is 15–50 days.
Symptoms are unusual in children and very common in adults (70%). Complications are rare; there is ~ 1% chance of fulminant hepatitis. Immune globulin (IG) is good prophylaxis only against HAV (use HBIG for hepatitis B). See Figure 1-6.
Diagnosis of acute infection: high titers of HAVAb IgM in serum (IgG indicates only a previous infection).

The incidence of hepatitis A has fallen dramatically due to immunization.
Hepatitis A vaccine (Havrix® and Vaqta®) is for use in patients 2 years or older, and given as 2 doses, 6 months apart. Virtually all of those completing the series develop protective levels of antibody to hepatitis A virus (HAVAb). Trends based on what is now known of the antibody levels suggest protection for up to 20 years in those who complete the series.
Indications for use of HAV vaccine:
• high-risk behavior
• children > 2 years old through age 18
• chronic liver disease
• travel in high-risk countries
• HAV vaccine is also given to all patients with hepatitis C; if these patients get hepatitis A, it can be fulminant.

Note that onset of jaundice is 3 weeks with hepatitis A and 3 months with hepatitis B—an important diagnostic clue!

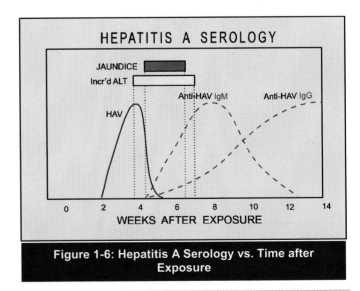

Figure 1-6: Hepatitis A Serology vs. Time after Exposure

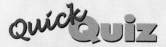

HEPATITIS C

Overview

Hepatitis C: Single-strand RNA virus. It is now one of the most common liver diseases in the U.S. [Know this section well!]. It is second only to NAFLD (Nonalcoholic fatty liver disease, see pg 1-48). Hepatitis C has blood-borne transmission, and had been the cause of 90% of transfusion-associated hepatitis prior to the early 1990s. Since then, especially with the 2nd generation HCVAb assays, the incidence of transfusion-related hepatitis has become very rare. Most HCV infections in the U.S. are genotype 1, which happens to be less responsive to treatment.

Hepatitis C genotypes are Ia, Ib, II, III, IV, and V. Genotype I is most common in the U.S. (> 70%). Genotypes influence response to treatment.

Those at increased risk for hepatitis C:
• especially IV drug abusers; common in prisons
• high-risk sexual behavior: with STD, sex with prostitutes, > 5 sexual partners per year
• blood transfusion before 1990
• tattoos, body piercing
• shared razors and toothbrushes
• snorting cocaine

The hepatitis C "rule of 2's":
• 2% of U.S. population
• 2% risk of needlestick transmission (though some say 5%+)
• 2% risk of neonatal transmission
• 2% risk of spousal transmission
• 2% cirrhotics with hepatitis C develop hepatoma each year

Chronic Hepatitis C

Whereas < 5% of adults with hepatitis B develop chronic disease, 70–80% of acute HCV infections become chronic! Hepatitis B has high virus counts, whereas hepatitis C has lower virus counts, as evidenced by hepatitis C viral RNA (units/mL).

These low virus counts are consistent with the more insidious nature of hepatitis C:
• Only 25% of acute infections are symptomatic.
• HCV infection has an increased likelihood to become chronic.
• The chronic form is relatively benign (25% are only carriers; 50% have no symptoms but have abnormal LFTs; 25% have chronic active disease with symptoms).
• Low rates of sexual transmission are seen in monogamous couples—2% after 10–20 years! This is low but it does occur—so safe sex is required! Sexual transmission increases with multiple sexual partners.
• Needlestick transmission from a known infected patient is 2–6%.
• Transplacental infection can occur (~ 2%), although this is only a little less than hepatitis B (5–10%).

70–80% of patients infected with HCV develop chronic hepatitis, and about 25% of these get end-stage cirrhosis after 20–25 years! And 1–4% of patients with cirrhosis develop hepatocellular cancer (HCC) each year.

Screen q 6 mo with alpha-fetoprotein and ultrasound for HCC (as with hepatitis B and alcoholic cirrhosis).

Chronic HCV infection has become the #1 cause of liver transplants in the U.S.

Vaccinate all patients with chronic hepatitis C against hepatitis A and hepatitis B.

HIV and Hepatitis C

In the U.S., 30% of patients with HIV are coinfected with HCV. These patients progress faster to cirrhosis than those with HCV alone. Best treatment of HCV for HIV-infected patients is combination therapy with pegylated interferon and ribavirin.

Extrahepatic Disease

Extrahepatic disease includes:
• small vessel vasculitis with glomerulonephritis and neuropathy,
• mixed cryoglobulinemia, and
• porphyria cutanea tarda (PCT).

Mixed cryoglobulinemia presents as a small vessel (leukocytoclastic) vasculitis with a rash consisting of "palpable purpura" or "crops of purple papules." Mixed cryoglobulinemia can result from chronic hepatitis B or C (in addition to various other occult viral, bacterial, and fungal infections).

PCT is associated only with hepatitis C (and not B). So, skin blisters? Think C!

notes

Serology and Hepatitis C

Tests:
- Within 2–4 months after an episode of hepatitis C, recheck for loss of HCV-RNA (PCR) to ensure that it has not become chronic. Note: This HCV-RNA test is not quantitative—but it is sensitive and can determine if there are more than 200 IU/mL of HCV-RNA present.

In a person positive for HCVAb, check for active virus with HCV-RNA. This is necessary because the HCVAb does not confer immunity (as does the HBV antibody to HB).

Treatment of Hepatitis C

Treatment of hepatitis C: If the patient has chronic hepatitis C and elevated liver enzymes, the current treatment is the combination of:
- pegylated INF-α (weekly injections—see hepatitis B), and
- oral ribavirin. INF treatment decreases risk of HCC.

Measure response to treatment by following HCV-RNA; if no response at 12 weeks—seen as a decrease in HCV-RNA by 2 log units—discontinue therapy. For those who respond, if the HCV is genotype 1, treat for 1 year; if it is genotype 2 or 3, treat for 6 months.

Notes on treatment:
Medications have no role in end-stage cirrhosis.
Ribavirin therapy can be complicated by hemolytic anemia but if mild, this is not an indication to stop treatment; rather, give epoetin (erythropoietin, recombinant). However, ribavirin is relatively contraindicated in cardiac patients with borderline hematocrit levels.
Caution using INF-α in the patient with a history of depression.

HEPATITIS D

Hepatitis D is an RNA virus that requires a coexistent hepatitis B virus infection for the hepatitis D to become pathogenic. It is usually found in IV drug abusers and high-risk HBsAg carriers. It usually does not make an acute HBV infection much worse but, if acquired as a superinfection in an HBV carrier, the infection is frequently very severe. If acquired acutely, HDV does not increase risk of chronic hepatitis B. Immunity to hepatitis B implies immunity to hepatitis D. Diagnosis: Anti-HDV IgM.

HEPATITIS E

Hepatitis E: single-strand RNA virus. Fecal/oral spread like HAV. Found in the Far East, Africa, and Central America, usually due to contamination of water supplies after monsoon flooding. Like hepatitis A, no chronic form is known. Unlike hepatitis A, hepatitis E carries a very high risk for fulminant hepatitis in the 3rd trimester of pregnancy—with a 20% fatality rate. With acute hepatitis in a traveler and negative standard serology (Hep A, B), think of hepatitis E.

HEPATITIS G

Hepatitis G is blood-borne, like hepatitis B and C. Mode of transmission is not well defined but is similar to HCV. There is evidence of infection in 1.5% of blood donors. It causes < 0.5% of community-acquired hepatitis. There is no evidence that HGV causes chronic liver disease.

CHRONIC HEPATITIS

Overview

There are quite a few causes of chronic hepatitis (see Table 1-12). We will discuss the causes in the same sequence as listed in the table.

Autoimmune Chronic Hepatitis

Autoimmune: Type 1 autoimmune hepatitis usually has an insidious onset and is most often found in young women. Type 2 is a childhood disease and will not be discussed. 50% of adult patients with autoimmune chronic hepatitis also have other disorders of altered immunity—thyroiditis, Coombs+ anemia, and ITP.

Autoantibodies are common; affected patients often have a positive ANA, anti-dsDNA, smooth muscle antibody (SMA), ANCA, and anti-actin.
The SMA test is the most specific of the autoantibody tests for type 1, and it is positive in ~ 80% of patients with type 1 autoimmune hepatitis. It is occasionally seen as an overlap syndrome with PBC or PSC. Refer to Table 1-8.
Anti-actin test is becoming available at many labs.
Early diagnosis is essential because this form of chronic hepatitis responds well to treatment. Other forms of hepatitis must be excluded, and the following autoantibody tests are done:

Table 1-12: DDx Chronic Hepatitis	
A	Autoimmune - ANA and SMA positive - Anti-actin positive - Anti-LKM-1 positive - Anti-SLA positive
B	Hepatitis B
C	Hepatitis C
D₁	Hepatitis D (only with Hep B)
D₂	Drugs (see text)
D₃	Diseases: - Wilson Disease - Alpha-1 antitrypsin - Hemochromatosis
F	NAFLD

notes

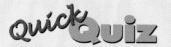
ANA, SMA, ANCA. You can also do antimitochondrial antibody—it is only occasionally slightly positive, but high titer occurs in primary biliary cirrhosis (PBC) and indicates an overlap syndrome. Remember, as a rule of thumb, PBC occurs in middle-aged women, autoimmune hepatitis occurs in young women. And PSC in middle-aged men.

Confirm diagnosis by characteristic changes found on histologic examination of a liver biopsy. These changes are charac-teristic but not specific, so drug history and serologic tests are required to rule out other types of hepatitis.

Treatment: Unlike other types of hepatitis, patients with autoimmune chronic hepatitis usually have a rapid reversal of symptoms and increased survival with prednisone +/- azathioprine.

Azathioprine (AZA) is used as a steroid-sparing drug. Initially, AZA has no effect as a sole agent, although, after a few years, some patients can be tapered off steroids and remain on AZA.

Alpha-interferon (IFN-α), although used in chronic hepatitis B & C, exacerbates autoimmune hepatitis and is therefore contraindicated.

Despite any response to the above treatment, there is no cure for autoimmune hepatitis, and it frequently progresses to cirrhosis and sometimes hepatocellular carcinoma (less often than with chronic viral hepatitis). Liver transplant is indicated for end-stage disease, although the disease process will slowly recur.

Chronic Viral Hepatitis

Chronic hepatitis **B**: Eventually leads to cirrhosis. There is a high risk of hepatocellular cancer, 1–4% (avg 2%) annually in patients with cirrhosis due to hepatitis B.

Medications used to treat chronic hepatitis B are shown in Table 1-11.

Chronic hepatitis **C**: Also eventually leads to cirrhosis. There is also a high risk of hepatocellular cancer, 1–4% annually in cirrhotics.

Medications used to treat: alpha-interferon and ribavirin. Combination interferon-ribavirin therapy for 12 months results in a 45–50% loss of genotype 1 HCV-RNA and 60–65% for genotype 2. See the acute forms discussed previously for more on these diseases.

Treatment of hepatitis C (alpha-interferon + ribavirin) significantly reduces the risk of hepatocellular cancer.

Again Note: Several months after an episode of hepatitis C, recheck for loss of HCV-RNA to ensure that it has not become chronic. After hepatitis B, recheck to ensure loss of HBsAg and HBV-DNA.

Also remember: Chronic viral hepatitis has the histologic characteristics of interface hepatitis with necroinflammatory changes and of fibrosis.

Drug-Related Chronic Hepatitis

Overview

Drug-related chronic hepatitis is associated with methyldopa, nitrofurantoin, acetaminophen, trazodone, phenytoin, methotrexate, INH (although INH far more commonly causes an acute hepatitis), and oral contraceptives. Histologic changes are similar to autoimmune hepatitis, and the patients are often ANA+. Hypergammaglobulinemia is also often present. Best treatment is to stop the drug.

Drug-related liver disease (acute) can be caused by the direct toxic, allergic, and/or idiosyncratic effects of drugs. Acetaminophen causes a direct toxic effect. Drugs causing an idiosyncratic effect are: halothane, phenytoin, chlorpromazine, and erythromycin. Drugs causing both toxic and idiopathic effects: methyldopa, INH (isoniazid), and sodium valproate.

Birth control pills, anabolic steroids, chlorpromazine and erythromycin are associated with cholestasis but not hepatitis.

Now let's talk a little more about acetaminophen, alcohol, methotrexate, INH, oral contraceptives, and aspirin.

Acetaminophen

Acetaminophen poisoning is discussed under Poisoning in the General IM section. Briefly, when acetaminophen is ingested, 90% of it is processed via the glucuronidation pathway, 5% is excreted unchanged in the urine, and 5% is oxidized by the cytochrome P-450 system. The P-450 system produces a toxic intermediate compound (N-acetyl-*p*-benzoquinoneimine, NAPQI), which is quickly reduced by glutathione. When there is an acetaminophen overdose, glutathione is rapidly depleted, and the resulting unreduced toxin causes direct liver damage.

Alcohol-acetaminophen syndrome: Chronic, moderate-to-heavy use of alcohol has a 2-fold effect: the cytochrome P-450 system is cranked up (i.e., more NAPQI is produced) and the amount of glutathione is decreased (so less is available for

notes

detoxifying the NAPQI). Therefore, long-time users of moderate-to-heavy amounts of alcohol who take acetaminophen in normal or higher doses are at risk for severe hepatic toxicity or liver failure.

Glutathione levels are depressed in malnutrition. Acetaminophen liver toxicity also may develop by not eating for 3–4 days (e.g., with an acute viral illness) and taking therapeutic doses of acetaminophen (i.e., < 4.0 gm/d)!

It has even recently been shown in healthy people taking the maximum recommended dosage (4 grams per day) for 2 weeks that 30% get an ALT > 100 IU/L!

Again, [Know]: Acetaminophen liver damage is potentiated with chronic alcohol use, one-time heavy alcohol use, malnutrition, chronic use, and even dieting.

Acetaminophen toxicity is the most common cause of fulminant hepatitis in the U.S. If suspected, draw acetaminophen blood levels; early treatment consists of using n-acetyl cysteine (Mucomyst®). There is also potential value to treatment if the diagnosis is made after 48 hours. Liver failure in this setting may be fatal or require lifesaving liver transplant.

Alcohol

Alcoholic liver disease results in a macrovesicular fat accumulation. There is also PMN infiltration in the liver. Women are more susceptible to alcoholic liver disease than men.

Alcohol induces GGT, so this enzyme is disproportionately high in alcoholic liver disease. Usually, there is a discordance between AST (SGOT) and ALT (SGPT) in this disease, with an AST:ALT ratio of 3:1. The AST is virtually always < 300—even with severe alcoholic liver injury.

Direct toxic effect is modified by other factors—including nutrition. Toxic effects may be additive. Alcoholics are very susceptible to acetaminophen liver damage because alcohol induces the cytochrome P-450 system (in most Board exam questions, acetaminophen is presented as an "over-the-counter pain reliever"). The combination may cause fulminant hepatitis.

Corticosteroids and pentoxifylline are of transient benefit in severe alcoholic hepatitis.

Certain drugs cause a similar picture—see NAFLD below.

Methotrexate

Methotrexate can cause an indolent, asymptomatic liver disease that progresses to cirrhosis.

INH

INH causes an occasional, mild, transient increase in liver enzymes. 1% of these develop a more severe hepatitis—the severity of which correlates with age.

Oral Contraceptives

Oral contraceptives (OCP) are associated with benign, hepatic adenoma, peliosis hepatis (blood-filled sinusoids), and focal nodular hyperplasia of the liver. So, young woman on OCP with a mass in the liver? Probably an adenoma. Hepatocellular cancer usually occurs in the setting of cirrhosis.

Aspirin and Reye Syndrome

Reye syndrome occurs exclusively in children < 15 years old. Although rare, it tends to occur after a recent viral illness—especially influenza A or B or varicella (chicken pox)—and especially when there has been concurrent ASA use. These patients get a fatty liver (microvesicular—as in acute fatty liver of pregnancy) and progressive encephalopathy. Elevated are ALT, AST, NH_3, and prothrombin time. Hypoglycemia, as a result of severe liver failure, is common. Mortality is 50%.

Amiodarone and corticosteroids are discussed below under NAFLD.

Other Diseases that Cause Chronic Hepatitis

The main diseases besides hepatitis that cause chronic hepatitis are Wilson disease, alpha-1-antitrypsin deficiency, and hemochromatosis.

Nonalcoholic Fatty Liver Disease (NAFLD)

Also called nonalcoholic steatohepatitis or NASH, NAFLD is an increasingly important cause of liver disease. NAFLD looks just like alcoholic liver disease, but there is no history of alcohol abuse. NAFLD is the inclusive term, which, like alcoholic liver disease, covers the spectrum of steatosis (fatty degeneration), steatohepatitis, fibrosis, and cirrhosis. 75–80% of "cryptogenic" cirrhosis is due to NAFLD.

The pattern of liver enzyme elevation is opposite that of alcoholic liver disease with ALT > AST.

NAFLD is associated with the following:
- obesity
- type II DM
- protein malnutrition
- hyperlipidemia
- amiodarone
- corticosteroids
- "DROP"
- prolonged IV hyperalimentation

DROP is a metabolic syndrome with: Dyslipidemia, insulin Resistance, Obesity, and increased blood Pressure. These patients with NAFLD and DROP have a higher incidence of fibrosis.

Treatment of NAFLD is not standardized. In general, treat with weight loss and control of any DM or hyperlipidemia. For patients with NAFLD and none of the common signs, recommend a low-fat diet. All patients with NAFLD should avoid alcohol.

HEPATOCELLULAR CANCER

Hepatocellular cancer (HCC, hepatoma): 75% have antecedent cirrhosis. HCC is associated with chronic liver disease of any type: chronic hepatitis B & C, hemochromatosis, alpha-1 antitrypsin deficiency, alcoholic liver disease, and autoimmune

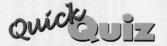

1) What is nonalcoholic fatty liver disease (NAFLD), and who tends to get it?

2) What are the treatment recommendations for NAFLD?

3) What disease is most probable in a patient with tender hepatomegaly, a RUQ bruit, bloody ascites, a high alkaline phosphatase, and a very elevated alpha-fetoprotein level?

4) Name the causes of cirrhosis.

5) Bleeding of esophageal varices is best correlated with what aspect of the varices?

6) What drug is used for prophylaxis against bleeding with large esophageal varices? What do you do with small esophageal varices?

7) What drugs and what endoscopic therapies are used for actively bleeding esophageal varices?

hepatitis. In addition, hepatomas are associated with aflatoxin (raw peanuts or raw peanut butter).

Alcoholic liver disease, frequently (75%) with concurrent hepatitis C, is the most common cause of HCC in the U.S. Chronic hepatitis B infection, acquired at birth, is the most common cause in developing countries.

HCC is associated with tender hepatomegaly, a bruit in RUQ, bloody ascites, and high alkaline phosphatase. 70–80% have a very elevated alpha-fetoprotein level.

Hypercalcemia and high hematocrit levels are indications of HCC-associated paraneoplastic syndromes and are clues to the diagnosis. Consider hepatocellular cancer in any cirrhotic who decompensates without an obvious reason.

Remember: IFN-α treatment in chronic hepatitis C reduces the risk of HCC.

For patients with cirrhosis from either HBV or HCV, do hepatoma surveillance with abdominal ultrasound and alpha-fetoprotein (AFP) levels every 6 months. Alternately, some places use helical CT or MRI—which are more expensive but have better sensitivity than ultrasound.

CIRRHOSIS

Overview

Causes of cirrhosis: Alcohol (most common cause in U.S.), hepatitis (B or C), post-necrotic (drugs and toxins), biliary disease, cardiac (from severe, prolonged right-sided CHF—which is rare), alpha-1 antitrypsin deficiency, hemochromatosis, Wilson disease, and schistosomiasis.

Complications of Cirrhosis
Esophageal Variceal Hemorrhage

1/3 of patients with esophageal varices bleed, and each bleed carries 1/3 mortality. With a bleed, the ratio of wedged:free portal pressure gradient is usually > 12 mmHg (normal ≤ 6), but chance of bleeding better correlates with the size of the varices.

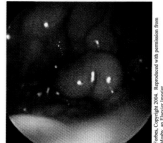
Image 1-28: Esophageal varices

Forbes, Copyright 2004. Reproduced with permission from Mosby, an Elsevier imprint

Prophylaxis:

Propranolol, with or without isosorbide dinitrate, decreases rebleeds and may delay or prevent the occurrence of the first variceal bleed. So, propranolol is given to all patients with large varices—whether or not they have bled.

Sclerotherapy is not good prophylaxis against the first hemorrhage—it actually appears to make things worse.

What do you do for the patient with cirrhosis and small esophageal varices? Do nothing—only big varices bleed!

Active bleeds:

Primary therapy of actively bleeding varices is endoscopic banding or sclerotherapy.

Somatostatin and its analog, octreotide, are splanchnic vasoconstrictors. These are frequently used in conjunction with endoscopic therapy and are a proven benefit over endoscopic therapy alone. Injection temporarily stops the active bleeding, allowing for good visualization for banding or sclerotherapy.

Vasoconstrictive therapy with somatostatin alone for acute bleeds is as good as sclerotherapy. But somatostatin has proven even better when used in conjunction with sclerotherapy.

Vasopressin, with simultaneous nitroglycerin (to minimize the vasoconstrictive side effect of vasopressin), has been used but is associated with more complications.

Balloon tamponade is rarely used anymore because it has a high rate of complications.

Any cirrhotic patient with GI bleeding should be carefully managed in the ICU. Consider elective airway intubation if there is active hematemesis, because aspiration pneumonia is common. Always do endoscopy. Remember: Cirrhotics can bleed from sources other than varices—like PUD. If the bleeding is due to varices, do endoscopic therapy with either banding or sclerotherapy.

All cirrhotic patients with bleeding varices or ascites are given prophylactic oral antibiotics to prevent spontaneous bacterial peritonitis (SBP).

Preventing rebleeds:

Propranolol is given to all patients who have had bleeding varices.

TIPS (transjugular intrahepatic portosystemic shunt) is used only for cases that rebleed. TIPS allows for decompression of the portal vein—effectively a portocaval shunt without the major surgery. The other main use for TIPS is for ascites due to cirrhosis.

Summary of treatment for esophageal varices:

• nothing for small varices
• propranolol for all large varices or any history of bleeding varices
• banding or sclerotherapy for active bleeds or to prevent rebleeds—preferably with somatostatin
• TIPS for rebleeds

Hepatic Encephalopathy

Hepatic encephalopathy may be precipitated by:
• GI bleed
• increased dietary protein
• hypokalemia
• tranquilizers
• azotemia
• constipation
• sedatives
• infections (pneumonia, bacteremia, urosepsis, and spontaneous bacterial peritonitis—SBP)
• alkalosis, which increases ammonia/ammonium ratio (NH_3/NH_4^+)—because only the non-ionized form, NH_3 (ammonia), crosses the blood-brain barrier. Acidosis has the opposite effect.

Signs of hepatic encephalopathy include fetor hepaticus (unique musty odor to breath and urine), hyperreflexia, and asterixis.

Treat with dietary protein restriction and lactulose. This disaccharide, more commonly used as an osmotic laxative, passes through the upper GI tract and is broken down by colonic bacteria into organic acids. The excess H^+ in the proximal colon:
• inhibits coliform bacterial growth and thereby decreases NH_3 production, and
• traps NH_3 as inactive NH_4^+.

Supplemental/alternative treatments:

Oral antibiotics (also to decrease NH_3 production) may be given if the patient doesn't respond to lactulose. Neomycin was previously used but has nephro/oto-toxicity. Metronidazole, rifampin, and vancomycin are now used.

Acarbose (used for diabetes mellitus) inhibits breakdown of carbohydrates into monosaccharides. Monosaccharides promote the bacteria that produce ammonia.

Probiotics alter gut flora and similarly decrease ammonia levels.

Hepatorenal Syndrome

Hepatorenal syndrome is also called "oliguric hepatic failure." The renal failure is caused by renal vasoconstriction during severe, decompensated cirrhosis. Usually fatal. Frequently iatrogenic—secondary to diuretics, NSAIDs, aminoglycosides, IV contrast, and paracentesis, or may be due to GI bleed or sepsis.

Know that urine sodium is very low in hepatorenal syndrome.

Current treatment: careful volume management and midodrine (an alpha-1 agonist) + octreotide (stimulates fluid absorption from GI tract).

PT in an Alcoholic

Again note: Alcohol causes malabsorption of some vitamins, including vitamin K. So, if the prothrombin time (PT) in an alcoholic is prolonged and is easily corrected by IM vitamin K, it is probably due to malabsorption—not liver disease (which affects more of the coagulation factors and is therefore harder to correct). Also, if a 1:1 mix corrects the PT, the disorder is due to decreased coagulation factors; if it does not correct, there is likely a circulating anticoagulant.

ASCITES

Causes

Causes of ascites are:
• cirrhosis
• CHF
• peritoneal diseases
• nephrogenic ascites
• pseudochylous ascites
• alcoholic hepatitis
• constrictive pericarditis
• myxedema
• chylous ascites
• fulminant and subfulminant hepatitis
• hepatic veno-occlusive disease (including Budd-Chiari)
• hypoalbuminemia (nephritic syndrome, protein-losing enteropathy, severe malnutrition)
• pancreatogenous (pseudocyst, disrupted duct)

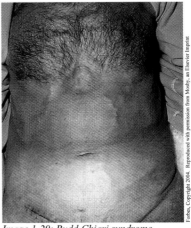

Image 1-29: Budd-Chiari syndrome.
Hepatic venous obstruction

Forbes, Copyright 2004 - Reproduced with permission from Mosby, an Elsevier Imprint

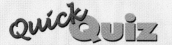
Cirrhosis-induced ascites: Ascitic fluid is resorbed via the peritoneal surface. Maximum capacity is ~ 900 cc/d. So, if you try to diurese off > 1 liter/day, it is at the expense of intravascular volume. This disease causes the most avid sodium retention state known.

Note: A chylous ascites is due to lymph blockage (trauma, tumors—especially 1° lymphoma, TB, and filariasis), not cirrhosis or CHF.

Diagnosis of Ascites

Determining the cause of ascites often requires analysis of a peritoneal tap specimen for appearance, cell count with differential, cytology, total protein, and albumin.

Know the following:

Appearance: Bloody suggests a tumor; cloudy, an infection; milky, lymphatic obstruction.

Cell count: If the cell count is elevated, do a C & S.

Chemistry: Portal hypertension is indicated by a serum-to-ascites albumin gradient (SAAG) > 1.1 gm/dL (i.e., low level of albumin in the ascites, usually < 1.0 gm/dL) and is seen in ascites due to:
• cirrhosis (most common),
• RHF,

Table 1-13: Causes of Ascites and Associated Findings

Protein and Albumin in Ascites		
Causes	(Serum) - (Ascites) Albumin	Ascites T. protein
Cirrhosis, liver failure, Budd-Chiari synd, myxedema, and SBP	> 1.1	< 2.5
Right heart failure	> 1.1	> 2.5
TB peritonitis, bacterial/fungal peritonitis, nephrotic synd, pancreatitis, and peritoneal carcinomatosis	< 1.1	> 2.5

• fulminant liver failure,
• Budd-Chiari syndrome, and
• myxedema.

A SAAG < 1.1 gm/dL (i.e., high level of albumin in the ascites and no portal HTN) is seen with ascites due to tuberculosis peritonitis, nephrotic syndrome, pancreatitis, and peritoneal carcinomatosis. Note: SAAG is a difference, not a ratio!

An elevated ascites protein level (≥ 2.5) is seen in all cases that cause increased levels of albumin. It is also seen in cardiac ascites! See Table 1-13.

TIPS (transjugular intrahepatic portosystemic shunt) is used to treat ascites caused by cirrhosis. As stated before, TIPS allows for decompression of the portal vein—effectively a portocaval shunt without the major surgery. A common complication is encephalopathy; therefore, it is generally not recommended for elderly patients who are most susceptible. As previously discussed, TIPS is also used in the treatment of rebleeding esophageal varices.

Spontaneous Bacterial Peritonitis (SBP)

Spontaneous bacterial peritonitis (SBP) is indicated by a peritoneal fluid with > 250 PMN/mL. Usual causes are *E. coli*, then *S. pneumoniae*, then *Klebsiella*.

Because SBP patients may not have abdominal pain or tenderness, you must consider SBP if there is a deterioration in the status of any patient with ascites, such as new-onset confusion, fever, signs of hepatic encephalopathy, or renal failure.

Risk factors for SBP:
• ascites protein < 1.0 gm/dL
• history of variceal bleed
• prior episode of SBP

These patients should receive either intermittent (preferred) or continuous prophylactic oral antibiotic therapy. Typically use oral therapy with a quinolone or TMP/SMX.

Rule out other causes of high WBC in ascites:
• Neutrocytic ascites: Basically this is PMNs > 250/mL with no evidence of SBP and negative cultures.
• Primary Bacterial Peritonitis (PBP) is due to perforated viscus. In cirrhotics, it can be confused with SBP.

Note that PBP has markedly different ascitic fluid abnormalities:
• protein > 1 gm/dL, frequently > 3 gm/dL
• glucose < 50 gm/dL
• WBC very elevated, often > 5000
• ascites fluid LDH > serum LDH

Active SBP is usually treated with cefotaxime (Claforan®). Milder cases can be treated with oral antibiotics.

IV albumin is also given in the treatment of SBP. Albumin maintains blood volume and thereby decreases the incidence of irreversible renal impairment and mortality.

notes

Treatment of Ascites

Treatment: mainly Na^+ and water restriction (needed only if the $Na+ < 125$). Then, if needed, start spironolactone, then a loop diuretic. Stop all anti-prostaglandin medications (e.g., ASA), because these decrease urinary Na^+ excretion! Also, do not give an aminoglycoside in this setting because it may precipitate renal failure.

Again: Do not diurese > 1 liter/d. It is okay to do daily paracenteses (up to 4 liters/d) during the initial treatment of recent-onset ascites or with severe refractory ascites if the patient's renal function is normal and there is:
• no GI bleeding,
• no sepsis, and
• no portosystemic encephalopathy (PSE).

With large-volume paracentesis, replace 8 grams albumin for each liter of fluid removed. Also, give albumin IV in life-threatening ascites, although it has only a short-term effect.

No longer used, the peritoneovenous shunt was limited by shunt failure and increased variceal bleeding.

HEREDITARY LIVER DISEASE

Review of Bilirubin

Hyperbilirubinemia is the main finding in hereditary liver diseases.

In general, only conjugated bilirubin passes the glomeruli and is excreted in the urine. The unconjugated bilirubin is tightly bound to albumin, and this complex is too large to pass through the glomerulus. Conjugated bilirubin is less tightly bound to albumin, and the 5% unbound portion easily passes into the urine.

So—bilirubinuria results only from conjugated hyperbilirubinemia. Because bilirubin is conjugated in the liver, bilirubinuria is an indication of cholestasis.

Table 1-14: Workup of Jaundice

	Acute Viral Hepatitis	Chronic Cirrhosis	Obstructive: CD Stone or Pancreatic Cancer
Bilirubin	≤ 20	≤ 20 unless impaired renal function	< 20
ALT/AST	> 400	< 400	< 400 usually
Alk Phos	NL-2xULN	NL-4xULN	4-10xULN
A/G	NL/NL	Low/High	Usually NL/NL
PT/PTT	NL/NL usu	High/High	Usually NL/NL
Cholesterol	NL	NL to Low	NL to High
Serologies A,B,C EBV, CMV	May be helpful	Excludes acute viral etio if needed	Excludes acute viral etio if needed
Abdominal US	NL	May be helpful	93/95 Sens&Spec if bili > 10 for 10 days

Unconjugated Bilirubin

Gilbert syndrome is a very common, benign, chronic disorder resulting in a mild, unconjugated hyperbilirubinemia. Remember: unconjugated = indirect = without bilirubinuria. The jaundice comes and goes, and is brought on by physical stress (especially surgery, exertion, and infection), fasting, and alcohol ingestion. ~ 7% of the population has Gilbert syndrome. It appears to be an autosomal dominant syndrome with variable penetrance!

Gilbert syndrome is due to decreased or absent glucuronyl transferase in the liver cells or decreased liver cell uptake of unconjugated bilirubin. 1/2 of patients have a very low-grade, chronic hemolysis. This probably reflects 2 separate syndromes but, for now, they are still grouped together. Phenobarbital stimulates glucuronyl transferase and decreases the bilirubin level.

Diagnosis: Increased unconjugated bilirubin after prolonged fasting. No treatment is needed.

Conjugated Bilirubin

If a patient is noted to have increased conjugated bilirubin after a major surgery, it is not Gilbert syndrome (which is unconjugated). It is most likely an entity called benign postoperative cholestasis. This is most often seen if the patient became hypotensive or required many transfusions during the operation.

Alpha1-Antitrypsin Deficiency

Alpha1-antitrypsin deficiency (autosomal recessive) causes a chronic hepatitis that eventually leads to cirrhosis. Diagnose with electrophoresis. Treatment: liver transplant—it does not recur in the transplanted liver!

Hemochromatosis

Hemochromatosis—2 types: genetic and acquired. Know: Multiple questions are likely about hemochromatosis!

The acquired form is usually from an iron-loading chronic anemia with 2° erythropoiesis, such as sideroblastic anemia or thalassemia and usually develops in men between ages 40 and 60 years.

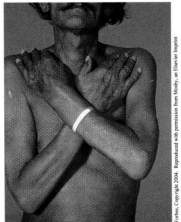

The genetic form involves the HFE gene and is autosomal recessive (AR).

In both types, there is abnormally increased intestinal iron absorption, which leads to iron deposition in the tissues. This iron deposition causes fibrosis and damage to organs—especially the liver, heart, pancreas, and pituitary.

Note: Symptomatic hemochromatosis is 10x more frequent in men—this is

Image 1-30: Hemochromatosis with slate-grey color of the skin, especially seen in the hands

Forbes, Copyright 2004. Reproduced with permission from Mosby, an Elsevier Imprint

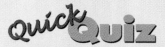

probably because of the effect menses has on iron stores in women.

Clinical findings:
- hepatomegaly (95%)
- gray hyperpigmentation (90%)
- secondary diabetes (65%), so suspect this in a 50-year-old with new-onset DM
- arthropathy (40%—esp 2nd and 3rd MCP joints!)
- cardiac involvement (15%)

Secondary hypogonadism also occurs and is caused by depression of the hypothalamic-pituitary axis. There is a 25–30% risk for hepatocellular cancer in patients with cirrhosis caused by this disease—higher than any other cause!

Diagnosis of hemochromatosis is suggested by high levels of serum Fe, ferritin, and transferrin levels. The most helpful screening test is transferrin saturation > 45% (you can read up on these lab tests at the beginning of the Hematology section). Liver biopsy confirms the diagnosis and allows for staging of fibrosis.

Liver biopsy is indicated for serum ferritin > 1000 ng/mL.

Confirm the diagnosis for the hereditary type with an assay for the HFE gene.

If this disease is successfully treated early enough—especially if cirrhosis is not present—patients have a normal life span with negligible risk of cancer. Initial treatment is weekly phlebotomies. Ultimately, the patient has phlebotomies 4x/year with the goal of a ferritin level between 50 and 100 ng/mL. This treatment results in decreased skin pigmentation, improved cardiac function, and prolonged life expectancy. But, if already lost, the secondary sex characteristics do not return (the damage is done!).

Wilson Disease

Wilson disease is an AR disorder that usually presents as liver disease or neurologic/psychiatric dysfunction in adolescents. It usually presents between ages 15 and 25. Other symptoms include arthritis from chondrocalcinosis. Wilson disease is

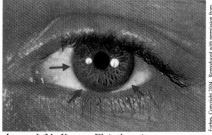

Image 1-31: Kayser-Fleischer ring.

caused by impaired excretion of copper into bile, which results in an excess copper in body tissues—especially the liver.

Hemolysis is common. Serum ceruloplasmin is low (in most liver diseases, it is high) and urinary copper level is high. Kayser-Fleischer rings are pathognomonic. These consist of a single brownish corneal ring, formed by copper depositing along the outer edge of the cornea. Liver biopsy confirms the diagnosis; it shows a high liver copper level (but remember, so do PBC and PSC!).

Screen for Wilson disease in all adults especially if < 40 years old with chronic liver disease without obvious cause. Screen with:
- serum ceruloplasmin,
- slit lamp exam, and
- urine copper.

All 3 of the above are positive in 25–30% of patients with Wilson disease.

Treatment is a 2-phase process. First, decrease copper levels, usually with chelation. Then maintenance therapy to prevent reaccumulation of copper.

Phase 1: Chelation with penicillamine (must give supplemental pyridoxine with this drug). If the patient cannot tolerate penicillamine, or has progressive neurologic manifestations, use trientine. Zinc is a 3rd option.

Phase 2: Maintenance therapy with low-dose penicillamine or trientine, or with zinc. Oral zinc blocks the absorption of copper. Low-copper diet is required (avoid nuts, peas, chocolate, mushrooms, shellfish, liver).

A liver transplant cures Wilson disease!

In fulminant Wilson disease, there is severe hemolytic anemia and a high serum copper level due to the release of copper from the liver. Penicillamine therapy is not effective; the only treatment is liver transplant.

LIVER DISEASE DURING PREGNANCY

1st Trimester

- Hyperemesis gravidarum can cause N/V, volume depletion, and mild increase in AST and ALT.

2nd Trimester

- Second trimester is best time for surgery for severely symptomatic gallstone patients.

3rd Trimester

- Remember that hepatitis E can cause fulminant hepatitis in the 3rd trimester of pregnancy—with a 20% fatality rate.
- Fatty liver of pregnancy is a very serious condition in which there is microvesicular fat deposition in the liver (as in Reye syndrome). There is only modest elevation of AST/ALT/Bili. It occurs in the 3rd trimester and is associ-

notes

ated with encephalopathy, hypoglycemia (again like Reye syndrome) preeclampsia, pancreatitis, DIC, and renal failure. Early delivery is required.
• Intrahepatic cholestasis of pregnancy causes itching and increased alk phos, bili, AST, and ALT.

LIVER TRANSPLANT

Consider liver transplant [know!] for almost all patients with irreversible end-stage acute and chronic liver disease. The selection process excludes many of these patients. The selection is usually made by a liver transplant committee at the liver transplant center. The process is inexact, and the waiting period for a liver is often more than a year. Evaluate patients with chronic, progressive liver disease early in the course of the disease.

The Model for End-stage Liver Disease (MELD) scale gives a fairly accurate short-term (3–6 month) prediction of mortality risk, and is used to determine organ allocation for liver transplant. It uses bilirubin and creatinine levels, INR (normalized prothrombin time), and etiology of liver disease in its calculation. The MELD score is:

$$3.8 \log_e (\text{bilirubin [mg/dL]}) + 11.2 \log_e (\text{INR}) + 9.6 \log_e (\text{creatinine})$$
$$[\text{mg/dL}]) + 6.4 (\text{etiology})$$
where etiology = 0 if cholestatic or alcoholic, 1 otherwise

Be sure and know this formula for the exam! And know the quick way to do logs without a calculator. (Just kidding ... on both counts.) Actually, all you might need to know about the MELD score is:
• < 10 = won't be on the transplant list unless has a liver tumor, and
• > 20 = candidate for transplant.

Common indications for liver transplant: Most types of chronic end-stage liver disease, metabolic liver disease, primary and secondary biliary cirrhosis, primary sclerosing cholangitis, and fulminant hepatitis. Cirrhosis with a small, early-stage hepatocellular cancer (HCC) is another indication.

Associated biochemical indications seen in end-stage chronic liver disease: Bilirubin 10–15 mg/dL, albumin < 2.5, and a PT > 3–5 sec above normal (10–12 sec). Other signs/symptoms suggesting it is time to transplant: Intractable pruritus, hepatic encephalopathy, bacterial peritonitis, intractable ascites, and the development of hepatocellular carcinoma.

Controversial: Using liver transplant to treat alcoholic cirrhosis.

Absolute contraindications: Preexisting advanced or uncontrolled non-hepatic disease, active alcohol or drug abuse, life-threatening systemic disease, metastatic cancer, and HIV infection. There are many relative contraindications, including advanced age.

A prior TIPS (see pg 1-49 under Complications of Cirrhosis) is not a contraindication to transplant. In fact, it is often a life-saving "bridge" to transplantation.

JAUNDICE

We've discussed many of the causes of jaundice in this section, and now I'll summarize these with a quick review of the workup of a patient with jaundice.

The actual differential diagnosis of jaundice includes:
• viral hepatitis
• drug-induced jaundice
• alcoholic liver disease
• chronic hepatitis
• gallstones and complications
• pancreatic cancer
• sickle cell disease
• Gilbert syndrome
• primary biliary cirrhosis (PBC)
• ascariasis
• primary sclerosing cholangitis (PSC)

...but the majority fall into the following 3 groups:
  1) acute viral hepatitis
  2) chronic cirrhosis
  3) obstructive problem (common duct stone or pancreatic cancer)

And these 3 causes are strongly associated with certain age groups:
  1) Acute viral hepatitis is the most common cause (85–90%) in those < 30 years old.
  2) Chronic cirrhosis is the usual cause (50–70%) in those 40–60 years old.
  3) Obstructive jaundice (common duct stone or pancreatic cancer) is the usual cause (80%) in those 60–80 years old without other risk factors.

If the patient is recently from outside the U.S., consider ascariasis. Especially if they have a high eosinophil count.

Workup consists of a careful history, ultrasound, and LFTs (see Table 1-14).

Ultrasound results determine the next test to be done:
• dilated ducts and stones: ERCP
• dilated duct to pancreas and no stones: think pancreatic cancer and do a CT
• dilated intrahepatic ducts: CT
• dilated ducts and ruling out PSC: MRCP
• if no dilated ducts: liver biopsy

NUTRITION

VITAMIN DEFICIENCIES

Time until onset of symptoms of vitamin or mineral deficiency—as when on TPN without vitamin supplementation (and barring other problems) [Know!]:

Weeks: Water-soluble vitamins, magnesium (muscle stiffness and cramps—often causes tetany in patients with Crohn disease), zinc (acrodermatitis and poor wound healing), and essential fatty acids.

notes

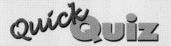

Months: Cu (hypochromic, microcytic anemia), and vitamin K (bleeding, high PT).

Year: Vitamins A & D (below), selenium (myalgias, cardiomyopathy, and hemolytic anemia), and chromium (glucose intolerance and peripheral neuropathy).

Several years: Iron, cobalt (anemia).

Many years: B_{12}.

These deficiencies are important. [Know them cold!] A good way to review this section is to fill in the following sentence, using the appropriate times, symptoms, and mineral deficiencies from above.

If, after 1–2 (_____), a patient on TPN develops (_____), you would suspect (_____).

More on vitamin deficiencies: Vitamins B and C are water-soluble, while vitamins A, D, E, and K are lipid-soluble. These will be discussed in this order. [Know all this info about vitamins and minerals!]

Vitamin B_1 is thiamine. Thiamine deficiency causes beriberi. It usually develops in alcoholics or in patients on chronic dialysis. There are 2 major manifestations of thiamine deficiency: wet beriberi and dry beriberi.

Wet beriberi: Symptoms of wet beriberi are heart failure, ascites, peripheral edema, and often an accompanying peripheral edema.

Dry beriberi: Confined to the nervous system (central and peripheral): peripheral neuropathy (symmetrical sensory, motor, and reflex loss), Wernicke encephalopathy (vomiting and nystagmus, ophthalmoplegia, ataxia, and mental deterioration), and Korsakoff syndrome (confabulation, poor recent memory and learning). Thiamine replacement usually cures Wernicke encephalopathy, but it reverses symptoms in only 1/2 of patients with Korsakoff syndrome—and only fully cures 25%.

Glucose infusions may precipitate Wernicke encephalopathy, so classic presentation is a closet drinker who develops ophthalmoplegia or nystagmus post-surgery. Always give thiamine to an alcoholic before starting an IV glucose solution.

Wernicke encephalopathy is a medical emergency. Immediately give thiamine 50 mg IM or IV. Repeat daily until the patient is able to take it orally.

Vitamin B_2 is riboflavin. B_2 deficiency almost invariably occurs in association with other vitamin deficiencies. Phenothiazines and tricyclic antidepressants increase the tendency to develop riboflavin deficiency. Patients present with a normochromic normocytic anemia, sore throat with hyperemic mucosa and glossitis, cheilosis, angular stomatitis, and a seborrheic dermatitis, especially involving the perineal/scrotal area. Symptoms are reversed with riboflavin.

Vitamin B_6 is pyridoxine. Deficiency is rare and usually caused by drugs, but may also be seen with general malabsorption syndromes and chronic alcoholism. The main drug culprits are INH, cycloserine, and penicillamine. Presenting symptoms include glossitis, cheilosis, vomiting, and seizures.

Vitamin B_{12} deficiency is discussed in the Hematology section (under Nuclear Maturation Defects) and Neurology (under Myelopathies). It results in a macrocytic anemia, smooth tongue, and subacute, combined degeneration of the spinal cord, causing initial pins-and-needles feeling, then decreased vibration and proprioception (position) sense and a stocking/glove decreased reaction to pinprick, and dementia.

Niacin deficiency causes pellagra. Niacin (nicotinic acid) is made from tryptophan in the body (so it is not actually a "vitamin"). Niacin deficiency is rare in the U.S. because niacin is now added to grains. It is still seen in carcinoid syndrome, in which tryptophan is used up, and when isoniazid (INH) is used in treating TB. Presenting signs of niacin deficiency are a dermatitis—especially on sun-exposed surfaces, glossitis ("bald tongue"), stomatitis, proctitis, diarrhea, and changing mental status, ranging from depression to dementia to psychosis (remember these by the 3 Ds—mucosal Dermatitis, Diarrhea, and Dementia). Patients may be hyperpigmented.

Vitamin C (ascorbic acid) deficiency causes scurvy. Ascorbic acid is a vital vitamin in connective tissue formation. Scurvy usually occurs in poverty-stricken urban areas. First symptoms are petechial hemorrhages and ecchymoses; then the patient gets hyperkeratotic papules around hair follicles, Sjögren syndrome, hemorrhage into muscles and joints, purpura, and splinter hemorrhages in the nail beds. In children, it affects bone formation and can cause intracerebral hemorrhage. Symptoms improve only when the normal pool is replenished (1.5–3 grams).

Vitamin A deficiency is a major cause of blindness in developing countries; night blindness is the earliest symptom of deficiency.

notes

Vitamin D deficiency causes rickets in children and osteomalacia in adults. Most vitamin D is synthesized in the skin (from a protovitamin D + sunlight), but some is absorbed from the gut. This vitamin D is then converted to 25 (OH)-D in the liver and further to 1,25 (OH)$_2$-D in the kidney—the active form of vitamin D. 25 (OH)-D is what is usually measured on blood tests. Vitamin D deficiency causes decreased absorption of calcium from the gut and decreased calcium resorption from the kidney. Deficiency also stimulates the release of PTH. Early in the course of the disease, the hypocalcemia is blunted by the increase in PTH, which increases absorption from the gut and also leaches calcium from the bones; so even though there is normal or slightly low serum calcium, the patient still gets the bone problems!

Symptoms in adults are often just musculoskeletal pain and weakness.

Main causes of decreased vitamin 1,25 (OH)$_2$-D:
- decreased production in skin: Elderly: Decreased skin synthesis at age > 70. Winter: Decreased sun exposure. Roughly 40% in northern climes are deficient at end of winter.
- decreased intestinal absorption: steatorrhea, insufficient dietary intake.
- kidney problem.

Consider vitamin D deficiency especially in any older patient who has musculoskeletal pain/weakness and especially if there is a history of fat malabsorption or the patient does not eat meats.

Vitamin E is an antioxidant. Deficiency is usually seen when there is fat malabsorption, and also a deficiency of the other fat-soluble vitamins. Deficient patients can have areflexia and decreased vibration and position sense, which is caused by deterioration of the posterior columns of the spinal cord. Intense research is underway assessing the antioxidant effects of vitamin E on atherosclerotic lesions.

VITAMIN OVERDOSE

Hypervitaminosis A can be caused by eating polar bear liver, but it is more commonly a result of over-ingestion of vitamin supplements, causing headache and flaky skin. A single massive dose causes abdominal pain, sluggishness, papilledema, and a bulging fontanel in infants. This is followed in a few days with desquamation of the skin and recovery. Chronic over-ingestion (25,000 U/day) is associated with arthralgias, anorexia, dry skin, hair loss, low-grade fever, and hepatosplenomegaly.

Vitamin B$_6$ excess can cause a peripheral neuropathy with normal motor and sensory function, but absent position and vibration sense.

Hypervitaminosis D results in increased calcium absorption from the bowel, hypercalcemia, and hypercalciuria. It probably increases the tendency for calcium renal stones. The hypercalcemia and hypercalciuria seen in chronic granulomatous diseases (such as sarcoidosis and lymphomas) are due to

an equivalent hypervitaminosis D state, in which there is increased 1,25 (OH)$_2$-D.

Vitamin E is relatively nontoxic. The main trouble with vitamin E is that large doses can cause a marked potentiation of oral anticoagulants.

Vitamin C megadoses increase the possibility of oxalate renal stones and can interfere with the absorption of B$_{12}$.

High doses of niacin can cause acanthosis nigricans and cholestatic jaundice. The flushing and pruritus often occurring at the start of treatment are prevented by taking aspirin 30 minutes before the niacin.

If the choice is between enteric feeding and TPN, enteric feeding is the better option. The glutamine and short-chained fatty acid substrates (fatty acids are manufactured in the small intestine) in the enteric feedings help maintain the integrity of the small intestinal wall—the loss of which is associated with the onset of multisystem failure. Glutamine is too unstable to be used in TPN. Percutaneous endoscopic gastrostomy is often used in patients who cannot swallow. It is a better alternative to the NG tube, and general anesthesia is not required. Contraindications to percutaneous endoscopic gastrostomy are delayed gastric emptying and gastric outlet obstruction. In these cases, various types of jejunostomy tubes can be used.

MALNUTRITION

Simple clues to malnutrition:
- weight/ideal weight < 70%
- lymphocyte count < 1000/mm^3
- low albumin or prealbumin
- low triceps skin fold thickness
- low urine creatinine to height ratio = (24-hr urine excretion of creatinine in μg) ÷ (height in centimeters) < 10 in men, < 6 in women.

Greater than 10% weight loss over 6 months indicates a possibility of malnutrition. Albumin is an indicator of nutritional status, but it may also be lower after major trauma or during an infection (due to vascular leakage of albumin or decreased albumin production by the liver). Malnourished patients are typically anergic. Triceps skin fold measurement is good only for long-term assessment of nutritional status. Short-term changes may not be meaningful because of changes in hydration and edema.

Indirect calorimetry units that measure oxygen consumption and CO_2 production are more precise and usually better for determining needed calories for in-hospital, critically ill patients.

notes

The following material is to assist you in integrating the information you have just reviewed in this section. These are purposely NOT Board-style questions since they are meant to cover a lot of material in minimal space. MedStudy does have Board-style Q&A products separately available in book and software formats.

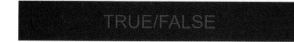

TRUE/FALSE

Note: for these T/F questions, follow along in the book section for clarification.

1) ERCP:
   A. High amylase after ERCP is usually an indication of acute pancreatitis caused by the procedure.
   B. ERCP is indicated in the workup of acute pancreatitis.

   [A=F, B=F (only if there are impacted gallstones or lack of clinical improvement in non-alcoholic acute pancreatitis).]

2) Esophagus:
   A. Achalasia results in decreased tonus of the esophagus and lower esophageal sphincter.
   B. In achalasia, the UGI shows a narrowing at the LES.
   C. Diffuse esophageal spasm is often precipitated by cold or carbonated liquids.
   D. Severity of symptoms correlates with tissue damage in esophagitis.
   E. Barrett esophagus is associated with squamous cell cancer.

   [A=F, B=T, C=T, D=F, E=F (adenocarcinoma).]

3) Stomach:
   A. Type A gastritis is the most common form of gastritis.
   B. Gastric cancer is usually an adenocarcinoma.
   C. The G cells make gastric acid.

   [A=F (type B is most common—80%), B=T, C=F (G cells make gastrin, which stimulates the parietal cells to make gastric acid.)]

4) PUD:
   A. Smoking decreases healing rate and increases recurrences of both types of PUD.
   B. Smoking does not increase the rate of perforation in PUD.
   C. *H. pylori* is the cause of virtually all gastric ulcers.
   D. In the workup of patients with a gastric ulcer, all should have endoscopy with at least 6 biopsy samples of the ulcer.
   E. With secretin stimulation, ZES patients have a paradoxical decrease in gastrin level.

   [A=T, B=F, C=F (most duodenal ulcers), D=F (this is done only with nonhealing gastric ulcers), E=F (paradoxical increase in gastrin level).]

5) Inflammatory bowel disease:
   A. Toxic megacolon is a complication of ulcerative colitis but not Crohn disease.
   B. Both prednisone and sulfasalazine are okay to give to pregnant patients.
   C. Azathioprine and 6-mercaptopurine decrease the relapse rate in Crohn disease.
   D. IBD is more common than colon cancer.
   E. IBD is the most common cause of bloody diarrhea.
   F. There is an increased risk of colon cancer in both UC and Crohn disease.
   G. Surgery is the cure for Crohn disease.
   H. Ulcerative proctitis is identical to early UC, but it has no increased risk of cancer.

   [A=F (both UC and Crohn's), B=T, C=T, D=F, E=F, F=T, G=F (colectomy cures UC, but not Crohn's), H=T]

6) Diarrhea:
   A. A 24-hour fast will stop all osmotic diarrheas, except possibly those from surreptitious ingestion of Mg-containing antacids. It will also stop secretory diarrhea due to fatty acids and fat malabsorption.
   B. If a patient with pseudomembranous colitis has a relapse soon after initial treatment, new therapy with a different class of antibiotic should be started.
   C. 3-day quantitative fecal fat is the best screen for malabsorption.
   D. Steatorrhea is defined as > 14 gm/d of fecal fat.
   E. A low xylose test is caused only by small bowel disease.
   F. Celiac disease is caused by gluten sensitivity and may lead to intestinal lymphoma.
   G. The small bowel biopsy findings in celiac disease can be mimicked by acute gastroenteritis.
   H. Some of the abdominal symptoms in Whipple disease are caused by lymphatic obstruction.

   [A=T, B=F (recurrence of the diarrhea is usually due to spores becoming active—so just repeat the same treatment), C=F (Sudan stain of the stool is the best screen for malabsorption, steatorrhea is the best indicator of malabsorption, and the 3-day quantitative test is the gold standard for diagnosis), D=T, E=F (many causes—see text), F=T, G=T, H=T]

7) GI Cancer:
   A. Small (< 2 cm) pedunculated adenomas are more likely to be malignant than large (> 2 cm) sessile ones.
   B. Hyperplastic polyps have only a small malignant potential.
   C. CEA levels are good for checking for intestinal cancer recurrences only if they were elevated before the surgery and decreased after the surgery.
   D. Surgery is the treatment of choice for all forms of intestinal cancer.

   [A=F, B=F (no malignant potential), C=T, D=T]

8) Pancreatitis:
   A. High lipid level may cause a spuriously low amylase level in acute pancreatitis.
   B. A pancreatic pseudocyst should be drained immediately.
   C. A plain film of the abdomen is useless in diagnosing chronic pancreatitis.
   D. In diabetes due to chronic pancreatitis, the patient is less susceptible to hypoglycemia.

   [A=T, B=F (surgical drainage is usually indicated if the pseudocyst persists > 1 month), C=F (if a plain film of the abdomen shows calcification of the pancreas, the diagnosis of chronic pancreatitis is made), D=F (much more susceptible).]

9) Hepatobiliary system:
   A. Cholelithiasis can be caused by hypercholesterolemia.
   B. Primary biliary cirrhosis usually occurs in middle-aged women, and ~ 35% of affected patients are antimitochondrial antibody-positive.
   C. Hepatic copper levels are elevated in PBC, primary sclerosing cholangitis, and Wilson disease.
   D. Primary sclerosing cholangitis (PSC) is more commonly seen in Crohn disease than in UC.

   [A=F, B=F (90%), C=T, D=F (PSC is strongly associated with colitis—so it is more often seen in UC).]

10) Hepatitis:
   A. Hepatitis B and C are transmitted by blood, while A and E are transmitted by the fecal-oral route.
   B. Immune globulin (IG) is recommended for prophylaxis against hepatitis B and A.
   C. Hepatitis B is the only RNA hepatitis virus.
   D. Hepatitis C causes 90% of transfusion-associated hepatitis.
   E. Hepatoma is associated with hepatitis B but not C.
   F. Alpha-interferon is the indicated treatment for autoimmune CAH.

   [A=T, B=F (IG for HAV, HBIG for HBV), C=F (HBV is the only DNA hepatitis virus), D=F (not since pre-1990's), E=F (hepatoma is associated with both HBV and HCV), F=F (Alpha-interferon is contraindicated in autoimmune CAH—it is indicated in the treatment of Hep B and Hep C chronic active hepatitis)]

11) Cirrhosis:
   A Not more than 1 liter/day should be removed by paracentesis.
   B. Alkalosis and hypokalemia are 2 precipitating factors for hepatic encephalopathy.

   [A=F (not more than one 1 liter/d should be diuresed off), B=T]

12) Hereditary liver disease:
   A. Rotor syndrome is similar to Dubin-Johnson syndrome.
   B. 99% of hemochromatosis patients have cardiac involvement.

[A=T, B=F (15%).]

ONE OR MORE CORRECT ANSWERS

13) A. Schatzki Ring.
    B. Diffuse esophageal spasm.
    C. Carcinoma.
    D. Peptic stricture.
    E. Achalasia.

1. 30-year-old with chest pain and intermittent dysphagia to solids and liquids.
2. 25-year-old with intermittent dysphagia to solids only.
3. Progressive dysphagia to solids and liquids, nocturnal aspiration.
4. Progressive dysphagia to solids only and a history of heartburn.
5. 75-year-old with progressive dysphagia to solids only.

   [1 (B) 2 (A-this often has intermittent SSx initially) 3 (E) 4 (D) 5 (C)]

14) A. Familial adenomatous polyposis.
    B. Gardner syndrome.
    C. Peutz-Jeghers syndrome.
    D. Juvenile polyposis.

1. No malignant potential.
2. 100% risk of cancer.
3. Hamartomas.
4. Adenomas.

   [1 (D) 2 (A,B) 3 (C,D) 4 (A,B)]

15) A. Hydrocortisone enemas.
    B. Prednisone.
    C. Sulfasalazine.
    D. Metronidazole.
    E. 6-mercaptopurine.
    F. Azathioprine.

1. Treatment of choice for mild UC.
2. Decreases relapse rate in Crohn disease.
3. Not effective in mild-to-moderate UC.
4. Treatment of choice for moderate UC.
5. Steroid sparing.
6. Causes reversible infertility in men.
7. Decreases relapse rate in UC.
8. Safe in pregnancy.

   [1 (A,C; also mesalamine) 2 (E,F) 3 (D) 4 (B—but not given long-term) 5 (E,F) 6 (C) 7 (A,B,C,E,F; also mesalamine) 8 (A,B,C)]

16) A. Gilbert syndrome.
    B. Dubin-Johnson syndrome.
    C. Crigler-Najjar syndrome.
    D. Rotor syndrome.
    E. Benign postoperative cholestasis.

1. Conjugated hyperbilirubinemia.
2. Unconjugated hyperbilirubinemia.
3. Occurs in 7% of the population.
4. Coarse pigment accumulation in the centrilobular hepatocytes.
5. Increased unconjugated bilirubin after surgery.
6. Increased conjugated bilirubin after surgery.

[1 (B,D,E) 2 (A,C) 3 (A) 4 (B) 5 (A) 6 (E)]

17) A. Wilson disease.
    B. Hemochromatosis.
    C. Alpha-1 antitrypsin.

1. Always hereditary.
2. Liver transplant is curative.
3. Low-serum ceruloplasmin.
4. Early treatment results in a normal lifespan.
5. May be caused by sideroblastic anemia or thalassemia.
6. Psychiatric dysfunction in adolescents.
7. Eye findings are pathognomonic.

[1 (A,C) 2 (A,C—but note that a patient with Wilson disease can
be maintained indefinitely on penicillamine or trientine) 3 (A) 4
(B) 5 (B) 6 (A) 7 (A)]

18) A. Hepatitis A.
    B. Hepatitis B.
    C. Hepatitis C.
    D. Hepatitis D.
    E. Hepatitis E.

1. High risk of fulminant hepatitis in third trimester of pregnancy.
2. Requires coexistent hepatitis B to be pathogenic.
3. Caused 90% of transfusion-related hepatitis prior to 1990.
4. No carrier/chronic states.
5. When concurrent with hepatitis B, is often fatal.
6. When acquired as a superinfection in a person with
   chronic hepatitis B, infection is often severe.
7. 5–7% go on to a chronic carrier state.
8. 60–75% go on to a chronic carrier state.

[1 (E) 2 (D) 3 (C) 4 (A,E) 5 (C) 6 (D) 7 (B) 8 (C)]

SINGLE BEST ANSWER

19) A. Ulcerative Colitis.
    B. Crohn disease.
    C. Both.
    D. Neither.

1. Patchy, transmural, deep ulcers.
2. Always starts in the rectum and spreads up.
3. String sign.
4. Cured surgically.
5. If skin lesions are present, they correlate with disease
   activity.
6. Associated with intestinal cancer.

[1 (B) 2 (A) 3 (B) 4 (A) 5 (C) 6 (C)]

20) A. Osmotic diarrhea.
    B. Secretory diarrhea.
    C. Both.
    D. Neither.

1. Isotonic.
2. $2[Na^+ + K^+]$ - serum osmolality > 50.
3. Bacterial enterotoxins.
4. Celiac disease.

[1 (C) 2 (A—osmotic gap > 50 = osmotic; osmotic gap < 50 =
secretory) 3 (B) 4 (C)]

21) A. Primary biliary cirrhosis.
    B. Primary sclerosing cholangitis.
    C. Both.
    D. Neither.

1. Usually occurs in middle-aged women.
2. Strong association with colitis.
3. Elevated hepatic copper level.
4. Antimitochondrial antibody-positive.
5. Anti-smooth muscle antibody-positive.
6. High bilirubin and alkaline phosphatase.

[1 (A) 2 (B) 3 (C—also Wilson disease) 4 (A—90%; occasionally positive in both autoimmune and drug-induced CAH) 5 (D—
this is positive only in autoimmune CAH) 6 (C)]

22) A. B$_1$ deficiency.
   B. B$_2$ deficiency.
   C. B$_6$ deficiency.
   D. B$_{12}$ deficiency.
   E. Niacin deficiency.
   F. Vitamin C deficiency.
   G. Vitamin A deficiency.
   H. Vitamin D deficiency.
   I. Vitamin E deficiency.

1. Major cause of blindness.
2. Wernicke-Korsakoff.
3. Carcinoid syndrome.
4. Phenothiazines and tricyclic antidepressants.
5. Hemorrhages into joints; splinter hemorrhages; petechiae.
6. INH.
7. Areflexia; posterior column deterioration.
8. Osteomalacia.
9. Glossitis, stomatitis, diarrhea, dementia.
10. Glossitis, seizures.
11. Heart failure.

[1 (G) 2 (A) 3 (E) 4 (B) 5 (F) 6 (C,E [oops—2 answers for this one!]) 7 (I) 8 (H) 9 (E) 10 (C) 11 (A)]

SHORT CASE SCENARIOS

23) A 40-year-old presents with a 3-month history of dyspepsia relieved by eating. No other symptoms. What workup is indicated?

[None; work up only if the symptoms persist on antacids and if the alarm signals are absent (see text).]

24) What are the 3 categories of dysphagia?

[1) Transfer disorders: e.g., CVA, ALS. 2) Anatomic or structural disorders: e.g., physical obstruction from cancer. 3) Motility disorders: e.g., disorder of esophageal peristalsis, lower esophageal sphincter spasm.]

25) Patient has a long history of dyspepsia and now has difficulty swallowing solids. What test should be performed now?

[Barium swallow for initial dysphagia workup, but then likely an EGD to check for probable peptic stricture.]

26) Teenager with acne presents with dyspepsia and dysphagia. What is the probable diagnosis? What is the workup? What is the treatment?

[Doxycycline-induced esophagitis; none; symptomatic treatment and stop the doxycycline.]

27) 70-year-old drinker with a history of progressive dysphagia—initially to solids and now to liquids. What is the initial test in the workup and what is the most likely diagnosis?

[EGD; cancer is most likely cause. Consider this in anybody > 65—especially if they are drinkers or smokers.]

28) 50-year-old with recent onset of epigastric burning pain. Normal CBC. Normal stomach acidity. Normal EKG. EGD found only gastritis. Is this more likely type A or type B gastritis? Is it likely to be associated with *H. pylori*?

[Type B; yes.]

29) A patient with Crohn disease is 3 months post-surgery, during which 15 inches of his distal ileum was removed. He develops diarrhea. What is the probable cause? How is it treated?

[This patient probably has bile acid–induced diarrhea, which is treated with bile acid sequestrants such as cholestyramine. When (roughly) > 100 cm of distal ileum is removed, steatorrhea results and a low-fat diet is started. Infrequently, medium-chain triglycerides are also used.]

30) A patient presents with a history of intermittent, frequent, loose stools for years. His stool has fecal WBCs and blood. C+S and O+P are negative on 3 stool specimens. On colonoscopy, mucosal inflammation from the rectum to the proximal sigmoid colon is found. What is the diagnosis? What is the initial treatment? What is used if the initial treatment doesn't work? Is this patient at risk for cancer?

[UC; oral sulfasalazine, oral or rectal mesalamine, or hydrocortisone enemas; prednisone; yes—colon cancer.]

31) 50-year-old patient has a 3-year history of chronic pancreatitis caused by ETOH. She had onset of smelly diarrhea 2 months ago. 3-day quantitative fecal fat was 60 grams. What is the probable cause of the diarrhea? What tests can be used to confirm this diagnosis?

[Pancreatic insufficiency; xylose absorption test, qualitative stool exam revealing undigested muscle fibers, neural fat, and split fat. The undigested muscle fibers indicate impaired digestion. It is further confirmed by a positive response to treatment with pancreatic enzymes.]

32) 50-year-old patient presents with 1-day history of fever, left-lower quadrant abdominal pain, and bloody stools. She has rebound tenderness in the area of pain. Which of the following is/are true?

   A. A sigmoid mass may be found on physical exam.
   B. The most likely diagnosis is the most common cause of GI bleeding in the elderly.
   C. The probable problem may cause colonic bowel obstruction.
   D. If not done previously, workup for colon cancer is required after symptoms resolve.
   E. All of the above.

[E]

33) A 45-year-old woman presents with complaints of fever and malaise for 2 weeks and jaundice for 1 week. She lives in a poor socioeconomic area. She says she last did IV drugs "a year ago." Blood tests show: ALT 1300, AST 1250, Bilirubin 4.5, Anti-HAV IgG positive, Anti-HAV IgM negative, HBsAg neg, HBeAg neg, HBcAg neg, Anti-HBsAg neg. Which of the following is/are true? More than one answer may be correct.

A. The patient has hepatitis A.
B. The patient does not have hepatitis B.
C. Hepatitis C is the most probable cause.
D. Primary biliary cirrhosis is the most probable cause.
E. None of the above.

[E. The patient does not have hepatitis A (otherwise, the Anti-HAV IgM would be positive). The patient may be in the "window" for hepatitis B studies; an HBcAb IgM should be done. Primary biliary cirrhosis may present with a high bilirubin, but the liver transaminases are not this elevated. Assuming that the patient is exaggerating the time since her last IV street drugs, hepatitis B is more likely than C. HIV testing should also be done.]

OPEN-ENDED QUESTIONS

34) What are 3 tests that may be used in the workup of GE reflux?

[If the patient is resistant to initial treatment or if there are alarm signals, then perform endoscopy. If the EGD is normal and the patient has refractory symptoms, then perform either 24-hour intraesophageal pH monitor or a Bernstein test.]

35) What is the most common connective tissue disease affecting the esophagus?

[Scleroderma.]

36) What endoscopic exams should a patient with pernicious anemia periodically have?

[None. Because the incidence of gastric cancer is so low, the 3xN increase in gastric cancer is not enough to warrant periodic endoscopic exams.]

37) Carcinoids often cause intolerance to what chemical?

[ETOH.]

38) With what 6 hypergastrinemic states is gastric carcinoid associated?

[Pernicious anemia, chronic gastritis, ZE, renal failure, hyperthyroidism, and vitiligo.]

39) Name the neurocrine, endocrine, and paracrine stimuli for gastric acid production.

[Neurocrine: vagus nerve; endocrine: gastrin; and paracrine: histamine.]

40) Which medication is preferred in patients with severe renal disease: sucralfate, H_2 blockers, or proton pump inhibitors?

[Of the drugs listed, sucralfate is preferred because it also binds $PO4$.]

41) What are the primary treatments for *H. pylori* infection?

[Usually triple drug therapy is used—2 antibiotics and a proton pump inhibitor. A good one with an eradication rate of ~ 90% is O-CLAM (omeprazole 20mg + clarithromycin 500mg + amoxicillin 1g—bid x 10d).]

42) Which is better (and why) for diagnosing cause of a UGI bleed—UGI or endoscopy?

[Endoscopy. This will find Mallory-Weiss tear, stress gastritis, and Osler-Weber-Rendu syndrome, which the UGI usually misses.]

43) A patient with a gastric ulcer also has achlorhydria after the stimulus of a meal. Is it likely the ulcer is malignant?

[Yes.]

44) What is stress-related mucosal damage, and what 2 classes of drugs are used to treat it?

[SRMD is PUD or gastritis associated with critical illness. Both antacids and H_2-receptor antagonists are effective treatments.]

45) Which extraintestinal manifestations of IBD do not improve with improvement of the colitis?

[Primary sclerosing cholangitis, uveitis, and ankylosing spondylitis.]

46) What are the prednisone-sparing drugs used in IBD?

[6-mercaptopurine and azathioprine.]

47) What are 2 important side effects of sulfasalazine?

[Leukopenia, and reversible infertility in men.]

48) Which drugs decrease the relapse rate in Crohn disease? Which in UC?

[The only drugs that decrease the relapse rate in Crohn disease are azathioprine, 6-mercaptopurine, MTX, and infliximab (for infliximab-induced remission), while all of the standard drugs decrease the relapse rate in UC!]

49) What is the "string sign"?

[In Crohn disease, the terminal ileum can become so edematous that the lumen is compressed and shows up as a string of contrast. The edema pushes the rest of the bowel away, so the "string" shows up well.]

50) Which inflammatory bowel disease is most likely to cause bile acid–induced diarrhea?

[Crohn disease (not UC) has problems related to disease/resection of the terminal ileum such as oxalate kidney stones, cholesterol gallstones, B_{12} deficiency, hypocalcemia (vitamin D malabsorption), bile acid–induced diarrhea (< 100 cm ileum removed), and low-bile-acid diarrhea (> 100 cm ileum removed).]

51) When is colectomy recommended for UC?

[Colectomy for UC is reserved for: 1) fulminant UC not responsive to steroids or antibiotics, and 2) if the patient has dysplasia in a mass lesion or high-grade dysplasia in flat mucosa.]

52) What is the difference between antibiotic-associated diarrhea and antibiotic-associated colitis?

[Antibiotic-associated diarrhea is a dysmotility problem, whereas antibiotic-associated colitis is pseudomembranous colitis caused by *Clostridium difficile*.]

53) In invasive diarrhea: Which is the most common type? Which causes joint aches? Which is seen in patients with sickle cell disease or with achlorhydria?

[Most common invasive diarrhea is caused by *Campylobacter*. *Yersinia* is associated with joint pains and rash. *Salmonella* is seen in patients with sickle cell disease or achlorhydria.]

54) Why are bronchial carcinoids more symptomatic than those in other sites?

[Bronchial carcinoids dump vasoactive mediators directly into the arterial circulation, causing more symptoms (flushing, hypotension, tachycardia, and explosive diarrhea.)]

55) What is the usual cause of diarrhea in an AIDS patient with weight loss and diarrhea but without fever? What are the other possible causes? With fever?

[If the AIDS patient has diarrhea and weight loss without fever, suspect *Cryptosporidia* (usual cause), *E. histolytica*, *Giardia*, *Isospora*, *Strongyloides*, and HIV enteropathy. Note: All of these organisms are noninvasive. With fever, think of *Mycobacterium*, *Campylobacter*, *Salmonella*, *Cryptococcus*, *Histoplasma*, and CMV.]

56) What are the 2 main etiologies of malabsorption, and how do you differentiate them?

[Malabsorption is caused either by decreased mucosal transport or by decreased digestion due to pancreatic insufficiency. They are differentiated by the xylose absorption test.]

57) If a patient has 100 gm/d of fecal fat, the diagnosis is _____. What will the results of the xylose absorption test show?

[Pancreatic insufficiency. Xylose absorption is not dependent on breakdown by pancreatic enzymes, so the xylose absorption test is normal in pancreatic insufficiency.]

58) Which other substances are absorbed similarly to D-xylose?

[The absorption of carotene, vitamin K, vitamin D, folate, and iron are also, like xylose, independent of pancreatic enzyme digestion.]

59) If you see a small bowel biopsy with foamy macrophages, what disease comes to mind?

[Whipple disease.]

60) At what age are the screening exams for colon cancer started? What screening exams are recommended that also screen for adenomas, and how often?

[Current screening recommendations for adenomas and cancer begin at age 50 for those who have no risk factors. The following may be used: flex sig every 5 years, colonoscopy every 10 years, double-contrast barium enema every 5 years, or CT colonography every 5 years. Start at age 40 if there is moderately increased risk (e.g., positive family history). With high-risk patients, use colonoscopy only; this is the best method for detecting colon cancer.]

61) What is the most common cause of small bowel obstruction? Of colonic obstruction?

[The most frequent cause of small intestine obstruction is adhesions. In decreasing order, the most common causes of colonic obstruction are: carcinoma, then diverticulitis, then volvulus.]

62) What is the most common form of intestinal ischemia?

[Ischemic colitis. Especially consider this in patients with CHF. Thumbprinting is seen on x-ray or BE.]

63) What physical exam technique allows you to differentiate between neurogenic and acquired megacolon?

[The digital rectal exam. In megacolon due to psychogenic constipation, the digital exam reveals a rectum distended with stool. In aganglionic megacolon, the rectal vault is empty!]

64) What is the usual course of a pancreatic mass in a patient with acute pancreatitis?

[A pancreatic mass in a patient with acute pancreatitis usually resolves—but it could also be a pancreatic pseudocyst, which, if it persists > 1 month, will probably require surgical drainage. Associated fever and shock suggest an abscess.]

65) What are the most common causes of acute pancreatitis? Of chronic pancreatitis?

[Acute pancreatitis: alcohol abuse and gallstones. Chronic pancreatitis: chronic ETOH ingestion.]

66) Name 7 causes of abdominal pain associated with an elevated amylase.

[Acute pancreatitis, acute cholecystitis, intestinal infarction, diabetic ketoacidosis, perforated ulcer, salpingitis, and ectopic pregnancy! Other causes of hyperamylasemia are increased salivary amylase and macroamylasemia (a benign condition due to a low urinary excretion of amylase).]

67) How should diabetes due to chronic pancreatitis be controlled—tightly or loosely? Why?

[Loosely. These patients are very prone to hypoglycemia because they no longer produce glucagon.]

68) What is the proper treatment for a patient with gallstones but no history of symptoms?

[No treatment is indicated.]

69) When is the HIDA scan used?

[The HIDA scan is best used for confirming acute cystic duct obstruction (i.e., acute cholecystitis).]

70) In which diseases is anti-smooth muscle antibody usually found, and in which is the antimitochondrial antibody usually found?

[Antimitochondrial antibody is seen in 90% of primary biliary cirrhosis patients. It is occasionally seen in chronic active hepatitis of both the drug-induced and autoimmune types. Anti-smooth muscle antibody is seen only in autoimmune CAH.]

71) Name 3 diseases with an elevated hepatic copper level.

[Primary sclerosing cholangitis, Wilson disease, and primary biliary cirrhosis.]

72) Primary sclerosing cholangitis has a strong association with what disease?

[Colitis—either ulcerative colitis or Crohn disease involving the colon.]

73) In what 2 diseases is fatty liver microvesicular?

[The fat globules are microvesicular in acute fatty liver of pregnancy and in Reye syndrome. All other types of fatty liver—from ETOH, protein malnutrition, AODM, obesity, or prolonged IV hyperalimentation—store fat in large cytoplasmic fat globules (i.e., macrovesicular).]

74) Which hepatitis viruses are spread by fecal-oral route? By blood?

[Fecal-oral: hepatitis A and E. Blood transmitted: hepatitis B, C, and D.]

75) How is a patient with hepatitis D virus infection affected if the patient is a hepatitis B carrier (vs. having an acute HBV infection)?

[Hepatitis D usually will not make an acute HBV infection much worse but, if acquired as a superinfection in a HBV carrier, the infection is frequently very severe.]

76) Name the "ABCDE" causes of chronic hepatitis.

[A: autoimmune; B: hepatitis B; C: hepatitis C; D: drugs; E: et cetera, which includes alcohol, alpha-1 antitrypsin deficiency, Wilson disease, and hemochromatosis.]

77) What is the treatment for chronic hepatitis B? For chronic hepatitis C?

[Alpha-interferon is the only medical treatment for the chronic active forms of hepatitis B and hepatitis C.]

78) What is a serologic marker for hepatoma?

[Alpha-fetoprotein.]

79) What is the treatment for esophageal variceal hemorrhage? What is given to decrease rebleed?

[Primary therapy for active variceal bleed is endoscopic sclerotherapy. Vasopressin with nitroglycerin is used if endoscopy is not available. TIPS (transjugular intrahepatic portosystemic shunt) is indicated if the patient rebleeds. Propranolol is prophylactic.]

80) In ascites, what does an elevated serum-to-ascites albumin gradient (> 1.1) indicate? In what types of ascites is there high ascitic fluid protein level?

[Portal hypertension is indicated by a serum-to-ascites albumin gradient >1.1 (i.e., low ascites albumin level) and is seen in ascites due to RHF, cirrhosis, fulminant liver failure, Budd-Chiari syndrome, and myxedema. An elevated ascites protein level (> 2.5) is seen in cardiac ascites, nephrotic syndrome, pancreatitis, tuberculosis peritonitis, and peritoneal carcinomatosis. With all except the first, the SAAG is < 1.1— (i.e., high ascites protein level).]

81) Name 5 factors that may precipitate hepatic encephalopathy. Does NH_3 or NH_4^+ precipitate it? Why?

[Hepatic encephalopathy may be precipitated by GI bleed, pneumonia, increased dietary protein, low potassium, sedatives, and also alkalosis, which increases ammonia/ammonium ratio (NH_3/NH_4^+). Only the non-ionized form—NH_3 (ammonia)—crosses the blood-brain barrier.]

82) If an alcoholic presents with bleeding and an increased PT, and if it is easily correctable by vitamin K, is liver disease the cause?

[No. The cause is malabsorption.]

MedStudy®

13th Edition

Internal Medicine Review Core Curriculum

Infectious Disease

Infectious Disease

Authored by Robert A. Hannaman, MD

With J. Thomas Cross, Jr., MD, MPH

Many thanks to *Infectious Disease Advisors:*

Alan A. Morgenstein, MD
Glendale, CA

and

J. Thomas Cross, Jr., MD, MPH
Vice President of Education
MedStudy
Colorado Springs, CO

Table of Contents

Infectious Disease

PPD 095 ID MKSAP.

CYTOKINES

Cytokines are produced by lymphocytes (which produce lymphokines), neutrophils, monocytes (monokines), and macrophages.

Interleukin-1 (IL-1) is a lymphokine historically known as "endogenous pyrogen," which mediates the generation of fever in the hypothalamus. IL-1 stimulates neutrophils to reproduce and congregate (chemotaxis), T cells to produce other lymphokines, and B cells to produce antibodies, and it causes fever! IL-1 also causes T cells to produce IL-2, which in turn stimulates the production of all the T cell types (helpers, suppressors, and killers).

Interferons: Another class of cytokines, the interferons, has 3 types: alpha, beta, and gamma. The most potent interferon in the immune system is gamma, which is produced by T cells (both helper and suppressor). Gamma interferon both decreases virus-infected cell proliferation and activates macrophages. Some macrophages also produce interferon. (Again: Macrophages and T cells produce interferon.)

Growth factor is the newer name that covers the interleukins, colony-stimulating factors, and erythropoietin. We now know that these substances are the actual molecules that combine with the cell-surface receptors and stimulate the cells. More in the Hematology section.

Many believe that unregulated cytokine activation is the origin of SIRS (systemic inflammatory response syndrome). SIRS may have an infectious or noninfectious etiology. When infection is suspected/shown, the condition is called sepsis. Tumor necrosis factor (TNF) may be the most important mediator. TNF is a cytokine released by neutrophils, monocytes, and macrophages in response to endotoxin (lipopolysaccharide; LPS). Once released, TNF amplifies the signal LPS and transmits it to other cells.

Drotrecogin alpha (activated; Xigris®) is an antithrombotic and antiinflammatory agent (recombinant form of activated protein C) that improves survival in patients with severe sepsis—i.e., Apache II scores ≥ 25.

NEUTROPENIA

Neutropenia (granulocytopenia) occurs in leukemia, bone marrow transplant, ablative chemotherapy, metastases to the bone marrow, and overwhelming sepsis. Previously, the most common infections in patients with neutropenia were Gram-negative, but this has shifted to Gram-positive organisms—probably due to the widespread use of 3rd generation cephalosporins and to increased central venous catheter use. Especially consider S. aureus and S. epidermidis. Gram-negative infections are still common. Corynebacterium jeikeium (JK) and fungi (Candida, Aspergillus, and Mucor) also may occur. The tendency for infection is directly proportional to the amount of granulocytopenia less than 500! If the patient is not neutropenic, but has a history of recurrent staphylococcal skin infections, recurrent lung infections, and lymphadenitis, suspect a granulocyte dysfunction.

If a neutropenic patient presents with fever, you must initially cover for Gram-negative organisms. Vancomycin or linezolid is usually added if any of the following are present: hypotension, mucositis, catheter-site infection, skin infection, history of MRSA infection or colonization, or the patient is clinically deteriorating. Antibiotics of choice in a neutropenic person with fever are:

- aminoglycoside with a beta-lactam; usually an antipseudomonal PCN (ticarcillin-clavulanate, piperacillin-tazobactam),
- antipseudomonal cephalosporin: ceftazidime (3rd generation) or cefepime (4th generation), or
- imipenem-cilastatin, meropenem, or doripenem.
- Also used, and some believe just as good, is a wide-spectrum beta-lactam alone—ceftazidime or IMP/cilastatin. Note that the ceftazidime has no Staph coverage.

If the antibiotics do not appear to be working after 5–7 days, add caspofungin (less side effects) or liposomal amphotericin B. Prophylactic antibiotics are not used. Although prophylactic quinolones have been shown to decrease the number of serious Gram-negative infections, they do not affect survival; so as yet, they are not used. Always start antibiotics in a febrile neutropenic patient immediately after blood cultures are drawn.

HUMORAL DEFICIENCIES

Humoral deficiencies (multiple myeloma, asplenia, ALL, CLL, and AIDS) are usually associated with infections caused by encapsulated organisms—especially pneumococcus, meningococcus, and Haemophilus influenzae. With acquired hypogammaglobulinemia (common, variable immunodeficiency), patients have recurrent sinus and pulmonary infections (often pneumococcus) and recurrent diarrhea (frequently due to Giardia). The rule of thumb: If a person has recurrent giardiasis x 3, check for humoral deficiency. Note that AIDS patients have a humoral deficiency in addition to the T-cell deficiency, because the decrease in CD4 cells decreases the normal suppressive effect that CD4 cells have on B cells, and there is an overproduction of nonspecific immunoglobulins—which "gum up the works."

The spleen is intimately involved with humoral immunity. Patients with actual or effective asplenia have the same infections as those with the above humoral deficiencies. Babesiosis and malaria are much more severe in splenectomized patients. This is easy to remember because babesiosis and malaria are similar in other ways—they are both intra-RBC protozoan parasites. Overwhelming Streptococcus pneumoniae infection is particularly associated with splenectomy.

IgA blocks viral attachment to mucosal surfaces, and IgG blocks viral attachment to host cells. Patients with IgA deficiency often have atopic diseases (asthma, rhinitis), are more susceptible to giardiasis, and some (those with associated IgG2 deficiency) have increased mucosal infections such as giardiasis, otitis media, pneumonia, and sinusitis—the last 3

notes

usually with encapsulated organisms such as *Strep pneumoniae* and *H. influenzae*.

COMPLEMENT DEFICIENCY

Complement—C1, C2, and C4—deficiency causes decreased activation of complement via the classical pathway. Although the alternative pathway takes up some of the slack, these patients still have recurrent sinopulmonary infections (and ear infections when young), caused by encapsulated bacteria. There also is an increased incidence of rheumatoid diseases—especially SLE! C2 deficiency is the most common deficiency in North American Caucasians; thus, consider this deficiency in patients with early-onset SLE.

C3 deficiency results in severe bacterial infections.

C5-C9 deficiency (late complement deficiency) causes infections similar to those in patients with humoral deficiencies or splenectomies—*H. influenzae*, pneumococci, gonococci, and meningococci. Know that patients with late complement deficiency additionally have a unique susceptibility to develop meningococcemia. Because of this, check any patient with meningococcemia for a terminal complement deficiency (~ 15% have it—check a CH50 or CH100). The complement cascade is discussed in the Allergy/Immunology section.

T-CELL DEFICIENCY

T-cell–deficient patients are said to have decreased "cellular" immunity. This can occur with:
- AIDS
- Hodgkin lymphoma if T-cell–derived
- T-cell variant of ALL
- corticosteroids
- post-organ transplant

These patients with cellular immunity deficiency are more susceptible to:
- fungi (including *Pneumocystis*)
- *Listeria monocytogenes*
- *Nocardia*
- *Mycobacteria*
- viruses (especially CMV and herpes zoster)
- protozoa (*Toxoplasma*)
- helminths (*Strongyloides*)

Transplant patients have decreased cellular immunity due to the required immunosuppressants. *Toxoplasma gondii* infection (pg 2-21) is usually due to a reactivation during immunosuppression. CMV (pg 2-27) is a very common infection 1–4 months after an organ transplant. Note: There is no increased tendency for infection with *Staph*, *Strep*, or Gram-negative organisms, although they still commonly occur.

More on post-transplant infections: As mentioned, these patients have decreased, cell-mediated immunity due to immunosuppressive drugs. Certain infections tend to occur in these patients during a fairly specific period of time after the transplant. [Know all the following!]

Table 2-1: Post-Transplant Infections (T-cell–deficient)	
Months after transplant	**Infectious Organisms**
0 to 1	Usual post-op nosocomial pneumonias and infections (Gram neg)
1.5	Herpes reactivation *Human Herpes virus 6,7 & 7 I V, M*
1 to 4	Protozoa (PCP, Toxo, *Strongyloides*), fungi, CMV, *Mycobacterium*, *Listeria*, hepatitis B, *Nocardia*.
2 to 6	Viruses (Varicella zoster, EBV, hepatitis C)
4 or more	*Cryptococcus neoformans*

- In the first month, the causes of infections are the usual nosocomial post-op bacterial infections. Another early infection is herpes simplex; HSV reactivates in 2/3 of seropositive transplant patients within 6 weeks of transplant! Provide prophylaxis with acyclovir or famciclovir.
- Between 1 and 4 months after transplant, look for the infections mentioned above for T-cell–immunodeficient patients. Especially consider: TB, *Listeria*, CMV (common), hepatitis B, *Nocardia*, *Toxoplasma*, and *Pneumocystis*.
- From 2–6 months post-op, viruses are the major infection. These include varicella-zoster virus, Epstein-Barr virus, and hepatitis C. *Cryptococcus neoformans* appears from about the 4th month onward. In transplant patients with symptoms of meningitis, include the CSF cryptococcal antigen test and/or India ink test in addition to the other CSF tests. See Table 2-1 .

Question: What previous infections or organisms might reactivate in a person with impaired cellular immunity? Answer: *Nocardia*, TB, *Cryptococcus*, blastomycosis, histoplasmosis, coccidioidomycosis, and *Strongyloides*. Also CMV and HSV.

Highlights:
Humoral – splenectomy – encapsulated organisms
Early complement – classical pathway – sinopulmonary infections with encapsulated organisms – C2 deficiency is associated with SLE
Late complement – encapsulated organisms – meningococcemia.
T cell = cellular; post-transplant; corticosteroids; and fungi, acid-fast, viruses, parasites.

notes: Polyomavirus BK does not cause meningoencephalitis.

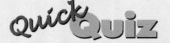

ANTIBIOTIC THERAPY

OVERVIEW

Review of Protein Synthesis

Most antibiotics work either by interrupting protein synthesis or cell wall synthesis (See Figure 2-1). First, let's review protein synthesis.

Protein Synthesis: Transcription

The DNA particle must be unwound from its supercoiled arrangement before it can be "read" by RNA polymerase. This involves cutting the strand, holding onto the cut ends to prevent them from being damaged, allowing the double helix to uncoil and the DNA to be copied, and then precisely gluing the cut ends back together again. The key enzyme that carries out this process in bacteria is DNA gyrase.

RNA polymerase moves along a section of DNA (a gene), uncoiled by the DNA gyrase and, following the coded messages on the deoxyribonucleotides, forms a string of complementary-paired ribonucleotides; i.e., a piece of RNA—more specifically, pre-mRNA. With the removal of an intron, the pre-mRNA becomes mRNA (messenger RNA). This is called transcription, because the DNA code is transcribed into a complementary RNA code.

Protein Synthesis: Translation

Ribosomes are the translation units that convert the coded message in the mRNA to a specific sequence of amino acids. A 30S ribosomal subunit attaches to the mRNA at the "ribosome binding site," then moves along it until it reaches the start codon (AUG). Here, a tRNA (with anticodon UAC) carrying an altered methionine (f-Met) binds with this subunit and mRNA to form the "initiation complex." A 50S ribosomal subunit then comes along and binds to this complex to form the 70S ribosome.

Amino acid-specific transfer RNAs (tRNA) attach to the 20 amino acids used in making protein. The bottom loop of these "inverted cloverleaf-shaped" tRNAs has 3 unpaired bases called anticodons.

As the 70S ribosome moves along the mRNA, tRNAs attach 1 at a time, bringing these amino acids with them. These amino acids are bound together, forming a gradually lengthening protein chain.

When the ribosome reaches the end of the coded message, translation stops. The ribosomal subunits then separate and detach from the mRNA, and the completed protein is released.

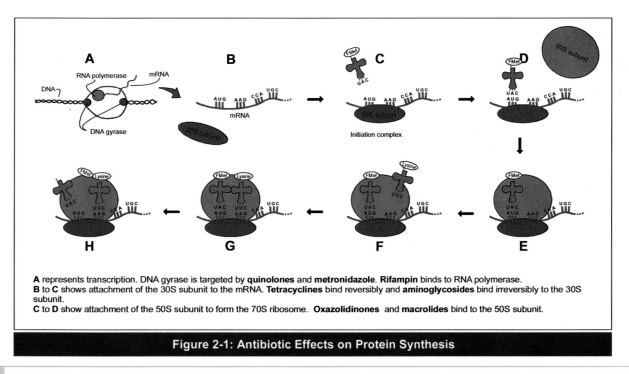

A represents transcription. DNA gyrase is targeted by **quinolones** and **metronidazole**. **Rifampin** binds to RNA polymerase.
B to C shows attachment of the 30S subunit to the mRNA. **Tetracyclines** bind reversibly and **aminoglycosides** bind irreversibly to the 30S subunit.
C to D show attachment of the 50S subunit to form the 70S ribosome. **Oxazolidinones** and **macrolides** bind to the 50S subunit.

Figure 2-1: Antibiotic Effects on Protein Synthesis

notes

Antibiotics that Block Protein Synthesis

There! Now we can see the effects of antibiotic interference with protein synthesis:

Rifampin binds to RNA polymerase and blocks initiation of the transcription of DNA to mRNA.

Quinolone antibiotics specifically target the DNA gyrase of bacteria. This allows the DNA gyrase to cut the double helix, but then prevents the cut ends from being rejoined.

Metronidazole, a very important antianaerobic and antiprotozoal agent, probably has a similar primary mode of action to the quinolones, although it also affects cell membrane function.

Aminoglycosides bind irreversibly (bacteriocidal) to the 30S subunit and prevent the 50S subunit from attaching.

Tetracyclines bind reversibly to the 30S subunit, distorting it so that the anticodons of the tRNAs cannot align properly with the codons on the mRNA.

Oxazolidinones are a new class of antibiotic of which linezolid (Zyvox®) is the first available. The drug binds to the 50S ribosomal subunit, thereby preventing attachment to the initiation complex.

Macrolides bind reversibly to the 50S subunit. They prevent peptide bond formation between the amino acids and, hence, keep the 70S ribosome from translocating down the mRNA.

Antibiotics Affecting Cell Wall Synthesis

Peptidoglycan is an exclusively bacterial polymer and is a component of bacterial cell walls. There is a variety of antibiotics that act at one or more stages of peptidoglycan synthesis.

Beta-lactams (see next) are a class of antibiotics that focus on attacking the cell wall. They contain a structure similar to that in the amino acids, which cross-link and stabilize the bacterium cell wall. Because there is no analogous structure in human cells, you can give these antibiotics at much higher doses without fear of toxicity.

Also:

To replicate DNA, folic acid is required. Bacteria are required to make their own folic acid from paraaminobenzoic acid (PABA). Trimethoprim and the sulfonamides block this process.

[Know]: Antibacterial agents must be 'cidal for effective treatment of endocarditis, meningitis, and infected neutropenic patients. Bactericidal antibiotics are the beta-lactams (PCNs, imipenem, and cephalosporins), fluoroquinolones, vancomycin, aminoglycosides, rifampin, and metronidazole. Bacteriostatic agents are erythromycin, tetracycline, linezolid, and clindamycin. Chloramphenicol is unusual in that it is normally bacteriostatic, but it is 'cidal against *H. influenzae*, pneumococci, and meningococci!

BETA-LACTAM ANTIBIOTICS

Overview

The first of the beta-lactam antibiotics was penicillin (PCN) and includes the semisynthetic PCNs (methicillin—no longer commercially available but remember it because of the nomenclature of MRSA and MRSE, oxacillin, and dicloxacillin), carbapenems, and cephalosporins. Because the bacteria rupture when the integrity of the cell wall decreases, these drugs are also bactericidal.

Penicillins

Penicillin, as noted above, has the beta-lactam ring. It is very active against meningococci, most streptococci (groups A and B, viridans group, and *S. pneumoniae*) *Pasteurella* (dog and esp. cat bites), *Listeria*, and many *Neisseria* species. It is also active against many anaerobes (such as *Clostridium*), but not *B. fragilis*. Know that even though PCN is indicated for meningococcal infections, rifampin or quinolones are better for eradication of the carrier state. Rifampin concentrates in the upper respiratory mucosa.

PCN is still the drug of choice for many infections:
- periodontal infections (but resistance increasing rapidly)
- erysipeloid   • group A and group B strep
- rat-bite fever   • yaws
- leptospirosis   • syphilis
- actinomycosis
- meningococcal meningitis and meningococcemia
- viridans Streptococci (some are now resistant to PCN and ampicillin)
- *S. pneumoniae* (PCN sensitive)

Ampicillin has a spectrum similar to PCN, but its spectrum extends to include certain Gram-negative rods—especially some *E. coli*, *H. influenzae*, *Salmonella*, *Shigella*, and *Proteus mirabilis*. However, it does not get *Klebsiella*, and many of the *H. influenzae*, *E. coli*, and *P. mirabilis* are resistant to it. Ampicillin is the drug of choice for:
- *Listeria monocytogenes* meningitis
- salmonellosis—if sensitive
- UTIs due to susceptible organisms
- enterococcal infections

Penicillinase-resistant semisynthetic penicillins, like nafcillin, oxacillin, and dicloxacillin, are needed against *S. aureus* because 85% have beta-lactamase (Note: Penicillinase is just a specific type of beta-lactamase). Unfortunately, there has been a rapidly expanding resistance in staphylococci to these (i.e., "methicillin-resistant"). Nafcillin is similar to methicillin, but it is not as likely to cause tubulo-interstitial nephritis (TIN; so methicillin is rarely used). These (nafcillin and dicloxacillin) are drugs of choice only for staphylococcal infections.

notes

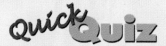

Note that nafcillin and dicloxacillin still can cause TIN. Remember that manifestations of TIN are ARF, eosinophilia, and WBCs in the urine.

Antipseudomonal PCNs (AP-PCN; ticarcillin-clavulanate, piperacillin-tazobactam) are better against the Gram-negative organisms (including *Pseudomonas*) and anaerobes (including *B. fragilis*). Like ampicillin—only better. They are the only PCN drugs effective against infections caused by:
• *P. aeruginosa* and
• *Acinetobacter*

Cephalosporins

Note:

Cephalosporins also contain the beta-lactam ring but are penicillinase-resistant. In general, cephalosporins have no activity against enterococci, *Listeria*, and methicillin-resistant staphylococci.

1st Generation

1st generation cephalosporins (cefazolin is the only one used much today) are active against most *Staph* (including the lactamase-producing strains, excluding the methicillin-resistant strains), and most *Strep*. No real anaerobic activity. 1st generation cephalosporins also get many of the community-acquired *E. coli*, *Klebsiella*, and *Proteus* (the Gram-negative coverage is superior to ampicillin).

1st generation cephalosporins are commonly given for:
• skin and soft tissue infections
• some surgical prophylaxis

2nd Generation

All 2nd generation cephalosporins are more active against the Gram-negative organisms (e.g., good against *H. flu*), and less active against Gram-positive bacteria.

Parenteral: Of the 2nd generation cephalosporins, cefoxitin (cefotetan is listed as a drug of choice in the April 2007 CDC guidelines for PID, but is no longer available in the U.S.) has variable activity against gut anaerobes. None of the 2nd generation cephalosporins consistently crosses into the CSF, so they are not used to treat meningitis.

Cefoxitin has good activity against *H. influenzae*, *Neisseria*, and Gram-positive organisms. It is among the drugs of choice for:
• PID
• abdominal surgery

Know that cefoxitin for the most part is used only for abdominal/pelvic infections because of its anaerobic coverage. The 3rd generation cephalosporins have largely replaced the 2nd generation except for this indication. Use cefoxitin as prophylaxis for GI and gynecological surgery.

3rd Generation

3rd generation cephalosporins are generally not degraded by beta-lactamase, and are especially effective against *N. gonorrhoeae* and *H. influenzae*. They also get most of the Enterobacteriaceae (*E. coli*, *Klebsiella*, *Proteus*, *Enterobacter*, and *Serratia*). They are not as active against *S. aureus* as the 1st generation. Of the cephalosporins, only some 3rd generations are active against *Pseudomonas*—especially ceftazidime (Fortaz®, Ceptaz®, Tazicef®).

Three of the 3rd generation cephalosporins can cross an inflamed blood-brain barrier, and so they are indicated as the primary therapy for meningitis caused by Enterobacteriaceae; these are ceftriaxone (Rocephin®), cefotaxime (Claforan®), and ceftazidime.

Remember: For empiric treatment of meningitis use ceftriaxone with vancomycin (which additionally covers resistant *S. pneumoniae*). For neonatal, elderly, and pregnant patients, add ampicillin.

There is emerging resistance to 3rd generation cephalosporins in many bacteria, so they are not recommended for routine treatment of community-acquired infections, except for community-acquired pneumonia (1st line) because they are good against PCN-resistant streptococcal pneumonia.

4th Generation

"4th generation" cephalosporin (cefepime; Maxipime®) is a broad-spectrum antibiotic with enhanced stability to cephalosporinases. It has the Gram-negative activity of 3rd generation cephalosporins and Gram-positive activity of 1st generation cephalosporins. It has limited anaerobic coverage. (1 + 2 + 3 = 4—it covers many of the organisms combined of the 1st through 3rd generations). Cefepime is useful in infections involving organisms with extended spectrum beta-lactamase (ESBL) production. This is becoming more and more important in nursing home and nosocomial infections.

Carbapenems

Imipenem is a carbapenem antibiotic that is very broad-spectrum. It is very active against *B. fragilis*. It kills most Enterobacteriaceae, *Pseudomonas*, and Gram-positive organisms, and is inhibitory for *Listeria* and *Enterococcus faecalis*. It also is effective against ESBL-producing organisms. The few organisms resistant to it include *Enterococcus faecium*, *Burkholderia* (previously *Pseudomonas*) *cepacia*, *Coryne-*

notes

bacterium jeikeium (JK), *Stenotrophomonas (previously Xanthomonas) maltophilia, Acinetobacter species,* and methicillin-resistant staphylococci (MRSA). Now, ~ 20% of *P. aeruginosa* are also resistant. Know that imipenem can lower the seizure threshold, so use it only as a last resort in seizure patients, or in patients with renal insufficiency.

Imipenem is always formulated with equal amounts of cilastatin (combo = Primaxin®). Cilastatin causes metabolism of imipenem to be blocked in the renal tubule, thereby increasing its half-life to 1 hour! Cilastatin has no effect on beta-lactamases.

Meropenem is a similar carbapenem with a longer half-life, so no need for an enzyme inhibitor. It is also less likely to cause seizures than imipenem.

Ertapenem is a newer carbapenem with once-daily dosing, but no activity against *Pseudomonas*.

Doripenem is the newest carbapenem and has similar activity and pharmacokinetics to meropenem.

Aztreonam

Aztreonam is a monobactam that is good only against aerobic and facultative Gram-negative bacteria. Its spectrum is similar to aminoglycosides and 3rd generation cephalosporins for Gram-negative aerobes. It is effective against most *Enterobacteriaceae* and *Pseudomonas*, but it is not active against Gram-positive cocci or anaerobes.

Beta-lactamase Inhibitors

Beta-lactamase inhibitors—sulbactam, clavulanic acid, and tazobactam—bind irreversibly to the beta-lactamase made by some bacteria. These inhibitors increase the activity of drugs against beta-lactamase–producing bacteria, such as *B. fragilis, Klebsiella,* and *S. aureus* (variably). Formulations:
• clavulanic acid + amoxicillin (Augmentin®, Amoclan®)
• clavulanic acid + ticarcillin (Timentin®)
• sulbactam + ampicillin (Unasyn®)
• tazobactam + piperacillin (Zosyn®)

OTHER ANTIBIOTICS

Vancomycin

Vancomycin is, in general, bactericidal. It is effective against most Gram-positive organisms, including methicillin-resistant staphylococci, *Clostridia,* and *Corynebacterium.* There are some vancomycin-resistant strains of enterococci and recent reports of vancomycin-resistant *S. aureus* (yikes!) *Staphylococcus haemolyticus* and a few *Staph epidermidis* are resistant (causing serious trouble in some endocarditis patients!).

Vancomycin sometimes causes the "Red man syndrome," which consists of tachycardia, flushing, occasional angioedema, and generalized pruritus. You can prevent this by either slowing down the infusion time or pretreating with antihistamines (but not H2-blockers). Previous formulations of

vancomycin had significant renal and ototoxicity; current formulations rarely cause toxicity in normal doses.

Daptomycin

Daptomycin (Cubicin®) is a cyclic lipopeptide active against Gram-positive organisms. It is the first drug to have bactericidal activity against *Enterococcus*. It has a long half-life and requires only once-daily dosing. It must be given IV. Generally, it is reserved for resistant organisms, such as MRSA and resistant *Enterococcus*. It is not effective for pneumonia because daptomycin is inactivated by pulmonary surfactant.

Aminoglycosides

Aminoglycosides are effective against many Gram-negative organisms. To be effective they require the aerobic mechanism of the cell, so they're no good against anaerobes. Aminoglycosides have a persistent, anti-Gram–negative effect after removal of the drug—known as the post-antibiotic effect! So, it is possible to dose aminoglycosides q 24 hours with equivalent or better results than the same daily dosage given more often. Once-daily dosing also results in fewer toxic effects. Because they irreversibly inhibit ribosomal protein synthesis, they are bactericidal.

Aminoglycosides are effective against *Yersinia pestis* plague (streptomycin), *Francisella tularensis* (streptomycin or gentamicin), *M. tuberculosis* (streptomycin), and *M. avium-intracellulare* (amikacin). Use gentamicin in combination with a beta-lactam antibiotic for the treatment of subacute bacterial endocarditis. You might also give gentamicin, along with rifampin, to prevent the rapid development of resistance to rifampin (as in prosthetic valve endocarditis). It is also given to febrile neutropenic patients, along with either a 3rd generation cephalosporin or an antipseudomonal penicillin.

Major side effects of aminoglycoside treatment are ear toxicity and kidney toxicity—these are more likely if either amphotericin B or cephalothin is also used!

Fluoroquinolones

Fluoroquinolones (ciprofloxacin, levofloxacin, moxifloxacin) are a set of very wide-spectrum antibiotics that inhibit bacterial DNA synthesis. They are very good against Gram-negative aerobic organisms—including rods.
Indications:
• Use ciprofloxacin, levofloxacin, and the newer agents for systemic infections.
• Fluoroquinolones are also good against all the usual causes of bacterial gastroenteritis (*Salmonella, Shigella, Campylobacter,* and *Yersinia enterocolitica*).

Fluoroquinolones are not effective:
• They are not good against anaerobes (*B. fragilis,* et. al.).
• Ciprofloxacin has only intermediate activity against Gram-positive organisms, including *S. pneumoniae;* hence, they are not a good choice for empiric treatment of pneumonia. (On the other hand, levofloxacin and moxifloxacin are alternative choices for community-acquired pneumonia.

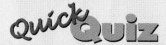

These fluoroquinolones are also effective treatment for atypical pneumonias).

• Do not use for MRSA because of the widespread, rapid development of resistance to them.

• Do not give to children (FDA says no one < 18 years of age; except ciprofloxacin is now approved for 2nd line therapy in children with UTIs) or pregnant patients.

[Know]: Some fluoroquinolones increase the levels of theophylline and cyclosporine by decreasing metabolism and increase the effect of warfarin by an uncertain mechanism. They do not increase the elimination of any drug. Although ciprofloxacin, like erythromycin, delays theophylline clearance, levofloxacin and moxifloxacin apparently do not.

Macrolides

Erythromycin is effective against *Mycoplasma pneumoniae*, *Chlamydophila pneumoniae*, *Campylobacter* (diarrhea), diphtheria, and pertussis. It is not so good against *H. influenzae* and is not effective against Q fever (*Coxiella burnetii*), which you would treat with tetracycline. Like the quinolones, erythromycin increases the effect of theophylline, cyclosporine, and warfarin.

Azithromycin has better *S. pneumoniae* coverage than erythromycin—and it has better *H. influenzae* coverage. It has a very long half-life (so, one/day dosage) and an intravenous form.

Rifampin is bactericidal. Never give it alone to treat an acute infection, because organisms rapidly develop resistance to it.

Ketolides

Telithromycin (Ketek®) is the first of the ketolide antibiotics, which are derivatives of macrolides. The drug has enhanced binding to the ribosome and so has activity against macrolide-resistant *Streptococcus pneumoniae*. Administer once daily. However, since its introduction a new black box warning has been issued as well as other warnings. It is absolutely contraindicated in patients with myasthenia gravis (causes respiratory failure) and has warnings of hepatoxicity, visual disturbances, and loss of consciousness. Now, it is FDA approved only for community-acquired pneumonia.

Oxazolidinones

Fluorinated oxazolidinones are an entirely new class of antibiotic that targets Gram-positive organisms, of which linezolid (Zyvox®) is the first available. Oxazolidinones have a unique mechanism of action for the blocking of protein synthesis. The drug binds to the 50S ribosomal subunit, thereby preventing attachment of the 30S+mRNA subunit—so, the 70S ribosome initiation complex is not made, and no protein is produced.

Linezolid is active against Gram-positive organisms, including MRSA (methicillin-resistant *S. aureus*). It is also effective against VRE (vancomycin-resistant enterococci) and anaerobes! Linezolid is available in oral (with 100% bioavailability!) and IV preparations. The oral form makes it a desirable alternative to vancomycin for MRSA—however, concerns of developing resistance and cost make this drug an unlikely 1st-line agent. In contrast, recent studies have suggested that linezolid may be superior to vancomycin for MRSA in pneumonia and soft tissue infections, but reports from Spain indicate that linezolid resistance is rising in MRSA. For the General IM Boards, vancomycin is still the current correct choice for empiric MRSA therapy, and they are very unlikely to ask you to decide between vancomycin and linezolid.

Linezolid can cause thrombocytopenia, anemia, leukopenia, and other signs of bone marrow suppression—especially if the patient has been taking it > 2 weeks.

Streptogramins

Quinupristin/dalfopristin (Synercid®) was the first of this new class of antibiotics. Its use essentially has been supplanted by linezolid (above). It was the first antibiotic approved for the treatment of serious infections with vancomycin-resistant *Enterococcus faecium*. The main side effects with this antibiotic are its severe myalgias and arthralgias. There is a high rate of thrombophlebitis associated with quinupristin/dalfopristin, so administer it through a central line.

Tigecycline

Tigecycline (Tygacil®) is the first of the new class of antibiotics called glycylcyclines, which are derivatives of tetracycline. It is a very broad-spectrum antibiotic with activity against Gram-positive organisms (including VRE, MRSA) anaerobes, and Gram-negative rods. It is not active against *Pseudomonas*. Give IV. Nausea and vomiting are its main side effects.

ANTIVIRAL AGENTS

Acyclovir is a nucleoside analog used for the treatment of herpes simplex and varicella-zoster viruses. Valacyclovir and famciclovir have similar indications.

Ganciclovir (previously DHPG) is used for the treatment of CMV infections in AIDS patients, especially for the chorioretinitis and colitis. Leukopenia is a side effect. Because it has only a suppressive effect against CMV, it usually needs to be given until the CD4 lymphocytes are > 200.

notes

Valganciclovir is an oral preparation with good absorption, leading to blood levels comparable to the IV form. Use it for acute disease or suppression of CMV. See pg 2-27 for more on CMV.

Foscarnet is used in patients with ganciclovir-resistant herpes infection, or as an alternative to ganciclovir for CMV.

Ribavirin is indicated for the treatment of RSV, and is used as part of combination therapy for hepatitis C.

Amantadine and rimantadine were effective against influenza A until 2006. See more on pg 2-28 under Influenza.

Oseltamivir (Tamiflu®—oral) and zanamivir (Relenza®—powder for inhalation) are neuraminidase inhibitors, a new class of treatment for influenza A & B.

See pg 2-32 for the antiretroviral medications.

ANTIFUNGAL AGENTS

Polyenes

There are 3 major classes of antifungal medicines: polyenes, imidazoles, and triazoles.

• Systemic polyene: Amphotericin B is the standard treatment for most systemic mycoses. Systemic amphotericin B is given IV only, and it has many side effects: fever, renal failure, phlebitis, acidosis, low K+ and Mg. Some recommend giving a test dose first. Every-other-day treatment is just as effective as daily dosage. Hypotension with the first dose may occur (decrease in peripheral vascular tone). Amphotericin B is associated with electrolyte abnormalities—especially hypokalemia, hypomagnesemia, and renal tubular acidosis.

• Lipid-associated amphotericin B preparations are less nephrotoxic but much more expensive. Use only when toxicity has become a problem with regular amphotericin.

• Topical polyene macrolides: Nystatin and amphotericin topical formulations are good only against cutaneous candidiasis (not ringworm). Both are also available in liquid form for oral and esophageal candidiasis.

Imidazoles

Systemic Imidazole

Ketoconazole for systemic use is given orally—increased gastric pH (low acid) decreases absorption. Food does not affect absorption. Ketoconazole does not penetrate CSF well. It is occasionally used for palliative treatment of Cushing syndrome caused by ectopic production of ACTH (i.e., cancer), because it blocks the 11-hydroxylase enzyme in the adrenal gland, thereby decreasing the amount of cortisol produced (more in the Endocrinology section).

Ketoconazole increases levels of indinavir and digoxin, and potentiates benzodiazepines. Side effects of ketoconazole include nausea and hepatitis. It also causes a decrease in androgen production, so patients may have decreased libido and males may get gynecomastia.

Ketoconazole is cheaper than fluconazole or itraconazole but has largely been replaced by them for serious fungal infections. Ketoconazole has many—sometimes dangerous—interactions with common drugs. Even though it is not used much anymore, the endocrine problems and side effects (gynecomastia) still appear on the Boards.

Topical Imidazoles

Clotrimazole and miconazole are available in both cutaneous and vaginal preparations. Other cutaneous imidazoles are ketoconazole, econazole, sulconazole, and oxiconazole. Other vaginal formulations are butoconazole and tioconazole. Spectrum and efficacy are the same. All are effective in the treatment of cutaneous candidiasis, tinea versicolor, and ringworm.

Triazoles

Systemic Triazoles

Itraconazole is a triazole analog of ketoconazole and is generally more effective and safer. The liquid formulation has much better bioavailability. Food enhances absorption. Indications are the same as ketoconazole (histoplasmosis, blastomycosis, coccidioidomycosis, esophageal candidiasis, and chronic mucocutaneous candidiasis), but also include aspergillosis, cryptococcosis, sporotrichosis, and onychomycosis.

Fluconazole (Diflucan®). Main side effect is N/V. A single 150 mg oral dose is effective in vulvovaginal candidiasis! Fluconazole is also effective treatment for oral and esophageal candidiasis and candidemia. It has excellent penetration into the CSF, and it is often used for maintenance therapy in AIDS patients with cryptococcal meningitis—after an initial 2-week course of IV amphotericin B. Fluconazole is the treatment of choice for chronic coccidioidomycosis.

Voriconazole is a new triazole with extended antifungal spectrum, including *Candida species*, *Aspergillus*, *Fusarium*, and *Scedosporium* (*Pseudallescheria*). The drug can be given orally or IV. Major toxicity is transient, reversible visual distortion and disturbance.

Posaconazole is the newest triazole with extended antifungal spectrum as listed for voriconazole, but also includes activity against *Mucor*. It is FDA approved for prophylaxis of *Aspergillus* and *Candida* infections in those with severe immunocompromised states, including prolonged neutropenia or stem cell transplant recipients with graft-versus-host-disease. It may be used for treatment of oropharyngeal candidiasis, particularly those refractory to itraconazole or fluconazole. It is an oral liquid agent that requires tid dosing.

Topical Triazoles

There is only 1 vaginal formulation: terconazole.

notes

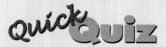
Other Antifungals

Other Systemic Antifungals

Flucytosine (5-fluorocytosine; 5-FC) is highly soluble and penetrates well into the CSF. Upon entering a fungal cell, it is metabolized to the antimetabolite 5-fluorouracil. If used alone, drug resistance develops quickly. For this reason, and because it may have a synergistic antifungal effect with amphotericin B, combine it with amphotericin B to treat cryptococcosis and serious forms of candidiasis. It can cause serious GI, hepatic, renal, and bone marrow toxicities—the latter usually presents as neutropenia and thrombocytopenia. Slight decreases in renal function can increase 5-FC to toxic levels.

Caspofungin acetate (Cancidas®) was the first of a new class of drugs called echinocandins—a glucan synthesis inhibitor. It is approved for invasive aspergillosis in severely immunocompromised patients. It now is approved for use in serious *Candida* infections. Caspofungin has no activity against *Cryptococcus*. It is the drug of choice for empiric antifungal therapy in febrile neutropenic patients.

Micafungin (Mycamine™) is a new echinocandin, which is similar to caspofungin but does not require a loading dose and seems to have fewer drug interactions.

Anidulafungin (Eraxis™), the newest echinocandin, has similar activity to the other agents.

Other Topical Antifungals

Undecylenic acid and tolnaftate are effective only against ringworm. The following cutaneous preparations have the same efficacy and clinical spectrum as the imidazoles: naftifine, terbinafine, haloprogin, and ciclopirox olamine.

ANTIPARASITIC DRUGS

Praziquantel (Biltricide®) is the only drug effective against all species of *Schistosoma*. It is also good against flukes and tapeworms (i.e., used to treat neurocysticercosis caused by the pork tapeworm, *T. solium*).

Albendazole is now used for cysticercosis and schistosomiasis. (pg 2-25)

Niclosamide is also used for the treatment of tapeworm, but it affects only those in the intestine.

Pentamidine, which is used for treatment (IV form) and for the prophylaxis (inhaled form) of *Pneumocystis jiroveci* (previously *Pneumocystis carinii*—which is classified now as a fungus), has many side effects, including azotemia (1/4), leukopenia, pancreatitis, and hypo- or hyperglycemia. It causes no significant skin reactions.

Nitazoxanide (Alinia®) is a newer drug approved for treatment of *Giardia lamblia* and *Cryptosporidium parvum*.

Antimalaria drugs: See pg 2-22.

VACCINES

For Vaccines, see "Preventive Medicine" in the General Internal Medicine section.

BACTERIA

GRAM-POSITIVE ORGANISMS

Staphylococcus

Staph aureus causes bacteremia, especially among IV drug users and dialysis patients. It is also a cause of toxic shock syndrome (TSS) and scalded skin syndrome (See Image 2-1). Pathogenicity (which is not the same as resistance to antibiotics!) is associated with production of entero- and exotoxin, coagulase, and leukocidin. In chronic carriers, *S. aureus* is found on the nasal mucosa cultures, but not usually in the blood.

The percentage of methicillin-resistant *S. aureus* (MRSA) infections has grown substantially due to indiscriminate use of methicillin and similar antibiotics. In most hospitals, 50–60% of *S. aureus* isolates are MRSA and, in some tertiary care centers, the percentage is > 50%! Unfortunately, MRSA is now frequently seen in community-acquired infections as well!

In carriers, it is difficult to eradicate. One can try a combination of topical mupirocin ointment (Bactroban®) and oral rifampin, but even then, it still recurs. In all cases of bacteremia and serious infection with MRSA, vancomycin is the only drug of choice on the Board exam (linezolid has become available, but it is very expensive and, in general, is not considered except in cases of vancomycin resistance; so, don't

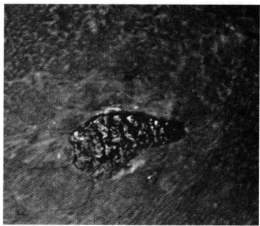

Image 2-1: Staphylococcal scalded skin syndrome

notes

use indiscriminately). Although other drugs may be used for their synergistic effect (gentamicin and rifampin), vancomycin is always required. In some skin and soft tissue infections, other antibiotics may be effective, including TMP/SMX or clindamycin, each +/– rifampin. There is rapidly developing resistance against quinolones.

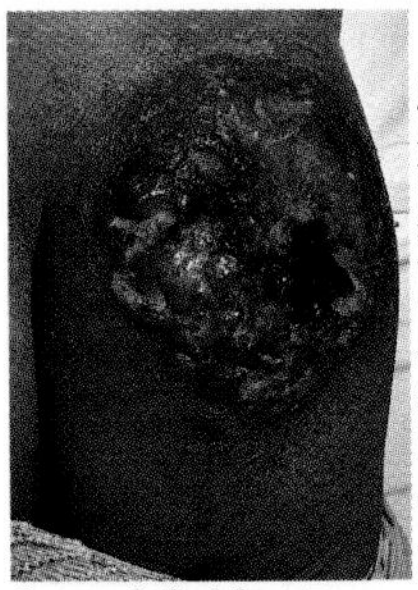

More on toxic shock: TSS often presents with red skin, hypotension, fever, diarrhea, and hypocalcemia. With young women, TSS is usually associated with menstruation and tampon use. A young woman with the focus in the uterus may have a bloody discharge or be menstruating. Do not treat the hypocalcemia unless either symptoms or ECG signs develop. Any time there is a post-surgical toxic shock, any device implanted during the surgery must be immediately removed (prosthetic device, implant, etc.)

Another cause of TSS is *Streptococcus pyogenes*. This usually results from a progressive skin infection—especially post-op and with chickenpox! Note: In *Staph* TSS, blood cultures are usually negative, whereas in *Strep* TSS, blood cultures are usually positive!

Staphylococcus is the usual cause of furuncles and carbuncles (See Image 2-2).

S. epidermidis and *S. saprophyticus* are examples of coagulase-negative *Staph*. *Staph epi* is almost always methicillin-resistant. It is the most common cause of both catheter-related bacteremia (catheter gets contaminated as it passes through the skin) and bacteremia occurring post-op when anything foreign was left in the body (e.g., prosthetics, including heart valves and joints, pacemakers, shunts, etc.). Treat with vancomycin +/– rifampin +/– gentamicin. *S. saprophyticus* causes UTI in young women.

Streptococcus

Streptococcus pneumoniae—Remember: You need functioning spleen and antibodies to defend against the encapsulated *S. pneumoniae* and *H. influenzae*—so both infections are seen more often in splenectomized patients (including those with Sickle Cell (SS) disease), very young and old patients, and in CLL, MM, and agammaglobulinemia (i.e., any antibody dysfunction or decrease). Alcoholics also are more susceptible, but not because of antibody problems.

~ 30% of *S. pneumoniae* have developed some degree of resistance to penicillin. For serious infections (e.g., meningitis or bacteremia), use ceftriaxone until you determine PCN sensitivity. For high-level resistance, use vancomycin for respiratory disease. A quinolone, such as levofloxacin, gatifloxacin, or moxifloxacin, also would be acceptable. For meningitis with high-level penicillin resistance, use ceftriaxone and vancomycin. For outpatients allergic to PCN, give doxycycline, cephalosporin, macrolide, or quinolone.

Remember: Post-splenectomy pneumococcal sepsis can be rapidly fatal, and can present with flu-like symptoms, purpura,

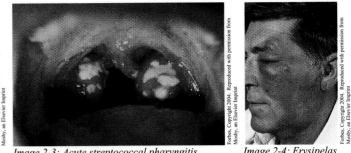

Image 2-2: Massive staph carbuncle

Image 2-3: Acute streptococcal pharyngitis

Image 2-4: Erysipelas of the face

and DIC (test question will have Howell-Jolly bodies on peripheral smear).

S. pyogenes is the only species in Group A beta-hemolytic *Strep*. It may cause strep pharyngitis (See Image 2-3), streptococcal TSS, rheumatic fever, erysipelas (See Image 2-4), or scarlet fever. The major protein on its cell surface is the "M protein." The M protein occurs in > 80 antigenically distinct types and defines which strains are rheumatogenic, cause glomerulonephritis, toxigenic for toxic shock syndrome, etc.

Strep pharyngitis (usually *S. pyogenes*) is more likely with each of these 3 findings: temp > 100°, tender cervical lymphadenopathy, and exudative tonsils. If none of these is present, chance of *Strep* is < 3%; 1 = 20%; 3 = 50%. Again: With *Strep* TSS, blood cultures are usually positive, whereas with *Staph* TSS, blood cultures are usually negative.

On the other hand, if a person comes in with tonsillitis, swollen cervical nodes, and fever but a negative strep test, do you treat with antibiotics? No! What else gives you these symptoms? Think upper respiratory viruses, mononucleosis—and don't forget acute retroviral syndrome (pg 2-36)!

Strep agalactiae (Group B) is seen in the very young and old, especially if the elderly patients are alcoholic or diabetic. It is a major cause of newborn pneumonia and meningitis. It is associated with UTIs in pregnant women, and it is also a cause of postpartum endometritis and bacteremia. It can originate from a GU reservoir. Treat with PCN or ampicillin.

Group D *Streptococci* are inhabitants of the GI tract and are causes of bacteremia and endocarditis. *S. bovis* is associated with colon neoplasm in ~ 30% of cases.

Enterococcus

Enterococcus faecalis causes 85% of enterococcal infections, while *Enterococcus faecium* causes 15%. The source of these organisms is usually either the GI or urinary tract. Suspect an enterococcal infection if a patient gets sepsis and/or endocarditis after a TURP.

All enterococci are resistant to all cephalosporins and penicillinase-resistant penicillins, and moderately resistant to the aminoglycosides. *E. faecium* is one of the few organisms resistant to imipenem, and is causing great problems with rapidly emerging, strong resistance to vancomycin ("VRE").

notes

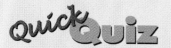
If sensitive, vancomycin, PCN, and ampicillin are only inhibitory. But...an aminoglycoside in combination with any of these is effective treatment. Therefore, you must treat sensitive enterococcal sepsis or endocarditis with vancomycin, PCN, or ampicillin in addition to gentamicin. Resistance to these antibiotics is increasing, so it is imperative that you do sensitivity testing.

Listeria

Listeria monocytogenes infections are associated with decreased cellular immunity syndromes, like AIDS, lymphoma, and leukemia, but they are also seen in neonates, the elderly, and pregnant women. For some reason, it is not actually seen as much as expected in AIDS patients. Mortality rate in listerial meningitis is 30% overall.

Like *Enterococcus*, *Listeria* is resistant to all cephalosporins (This is why you include ampicillin in the empiric treatment for meningitis in the elderly or neonates). Also, as with the enterococci, PCN and ampicillin are only inhibitory. But... an aminoglycoside in combination with either of these is very effective treatment.

Even so, most mild-to-moderate cases of listeriosis do not require an aminoglycoside, but treat resistant or serious cases with PCN or ampicillin in combination with an aminoglycoside. Vancomycin or TMP/SMX if allergic to PCN. Because aminoglycosides do not penetrate the CSF well, use very high-dose PCN or ampicillin to treat listerial meningitis. Again:

• Mild-to-moderate listeriosis: Ampicillin
• Serious/resistant: Amp + aminoglycoside
• Listerial meningitis: high-dose Amp +/- aminoglycoside

Corynebacterium diphtheriae, JK, and Arcanobacterium hemolyticum

Corynebacterium diphtheriae causes **diphtheria** (See Image 2-5). Diphtheria is an upper respiratory infection with a gray-white **pharyngeal membrane** (See Image 2-6), hoarseness, sore throat, and a low fever (< 101°). Low fever! Toxic effects include myocarditis with possible cardiac failure and polyneuritis. Treatment is erythromycin. Second choice is penicillin. Diphtheria antitoxin is always given with the antibiotic.

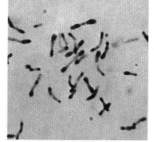

Image 2-5: C. diphtheriae

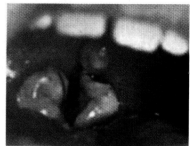

Image 2-6: Pharyngeal membrane

Corynebacterium jeikeium
(JK) is especially a problem in neutropenic patients and in bone marrow transplant units, where it is a cause of IV catheter-related infections. It is resistant to most drugs. Vancomycin is the only effective agent.

Arcanobacterium haemolyticum (previously *Corynebacterium haemolyticum*) causes pharyngitis in adolescents, similar to that of *Strep pyogenes*, with a desquamative scarlatiniform rash and lymphadenitis. Treat with PCN, erythromycin, or tetracycline.

Bacillus anthracis and Bacillus cereus

Bacillus anthracis are large, Gram-positive rods (bacilli) that cause **anthrax [Know!]**. There are 3 main clinical manifestations: cutaneous (95%), pulmonic ("woolsorters disease"), and pharyngeal + gastrointestinal. Inoculation occurs from handling contaminated hides/wool or (more recently) maliciously contaminated sources such as mail, or eating contaminated meat. Virulence requires a 3-component protein exotoxin. The component proteins are edema factor (causes edema), lethal factor (causes death!), and "protective antigen." Anthrax is not contagious.

Cutaneous anthrax starts as a **painless** papule that vesiculates and forms a **painless** ulcer (See Image 2-7), then a **painless**

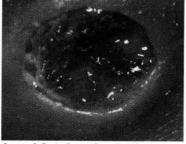

Image 2-7: Anthrax ulcer (painless)

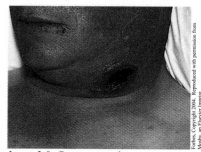

Image 2-8: Cutaneous anthrax

notes

black eschar, often with a lot of nonpitting, painless induration and swelling (See Image 2-8).

Inhalation anthrax presents similarly to influenza with malaise, fever, and myalgias. After 2–3 days, there is a dramatic worsening of symptoms with hypoxia and then hypotension and death. An important diagnostic finding is mediastinal widening.

Gastrointestinal anthrax is acquired by eating undercooked contaminated meat. Patients get pharyngeal eschars and/ or severe GI distress.

Anthrax is usually sensitive to penicillin, tetracycline, erythromycin, and to quinolones. The recent anthrax bioterrorism infections in the U.S. had an inducible beta-lactamase, which led to the recommendation of the quinolones for its treatment and prophylaxis.

Bacillus cereus is a close relative of *Bacillus anthracis*. Emetic-toxin and enterotoxin-producing strains cause gastroenteritis of 2 varieties:

1) a short incubation (1–6 hr) emetic type, and
2) a longer incubation (8–16 hr) diarrheal type.

Like *S. aureus*, the emetic toxin is produced outside the host, is preformed in foods, and therefore provokes a quick onset of symptoms (1–6 hr). The emetic form is associated with fried rice left too long at room temperature. This gastroenteritis is self-limited and necessitates only symptomatic treatment.

The diarrheal form can be from preformed enterotoxins or produced *in vivo* in the human intestine after the ingestion of the bacilli. It results in a profuse, watery, non-bloody diarrhea, accompanied by abdominal pain and cramps, nausea and occasionally vomiting. The incubation period is 8–16 hours, and it resembles *C. perfringens* food poisoning (see below). Symptoms usually resolve in 12–24 hours. No specific therapy is necessary.

B. cereus is an occasional cause of infection in contact lens wearers, after a traumatic eye injury, and is a possible cause of IV catheter-related infections. Treatment for serious disease is vancomycin.

Clostridium

Clostridium is a strict anaerobic Gram-positive rod [Know]:

- *C. difficile* causes antibiotic-associated colitis (see pg 2-43).
- *C. botulinum* causes botulism—this toxin is the most potent known! It blocks presynaptic acetylcholine release.
- *C. perfringens* is one of the most common causes of food poisoning in the U.S. and presents as a 24-hour (or less) diarrheal illness. It is associated with contaminated meat or gravy.
- *C. septicum*: The majority of patients with *C. septicum* sepsis have an associated GI malignancy!
- *C. tetani* is the cause of tetanus.

Cellulitis and gas gangrene (See Image 2-9) can be caused by *C. septicum, perfringens, tetani*, or *novyi*. The main toxin in all *Clostridia* is the "alpha toxin." For acute antibiotic treatment of *C. tetani*, metronidazole is now the drug of choice instead of PCN, which is still an alternative. For tetanus, also

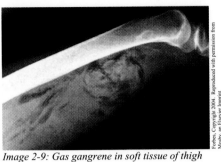

Image 2-9: Gas gangrene in soft tissue of thigh after penetrating injury

remember to use tetanus toxoid and tetanus immune globulin! Look for it in an elderly person with lockjaw!

GRAM-NEGATIVE BACTERIA

Neisseria

Neisseria meningitidis is a Gram-negative coccus that is an occasional, ordinary inhabitant of the human throat. It usually does not cause disease, because specific antibodies (humoral defense) and complement lyse the organisms as they enter the bloodstream.

Patients with complement deficiency are especially prone to meningococcemia. Meningococcemia presents with fever, hypotension, diffuse purpuric lesions, and DIC (See Image 2-10). For more on DIC, see Hematology section.

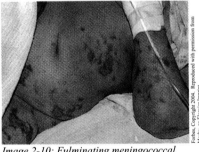

Image 2-10: Fulminating meningococcal septicemia

Penicillin G is the treatment of choice; for the penicillin-allergic, give fluoroquinolones (to adults) or 3rd generation cephalosporins (if rash only) to child. With prompt treatment, the mortality rate of meningococcemia is 10%. Rifampin or fluoroquinolones are better for eradicating the carrier state because they concentrate in the throat mucosa.

Neisseria gonorrhoeae is a common cause of sexually transmitted disease. It is a Gram-negative organism that is usually found as diplococci. The penicillinase-producing strains of *N. gonorrhoeae* now account for 80% of cases in many areas in Asia and Africa, and are also common in the U.S. More on pg 2-44.

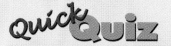

1) Which organism causes the "Chinese fried-rice" syndrome of gastrointestinal upset?

2) Which Clostridium species causes botulism? Colitis? Food poisoning?

3) Which Clostridium species is associated with gastrointestinal malignancy?

4) What organism should you strongly consider responsible for diarrhea if an "iguana" is mentioned in the patient's history?

5) What is a good way to confirm a diagnosis of bubonic plague? ("from a distance" is not correct!)

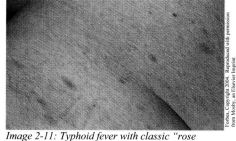

Image 2-11: Typhoid fever with classic "rose spots"

Moraxella

Moraxella catarrhalis (formerly *Branhamella catarrhalis* [formerly *Neisseria catarrhalis*!]) is a Gram-negative coccus that causes respiratory infections, especially in immunodeficient patients and patients with COPD. It is a common cause of sinusitis in adults and otitis media in children. Treat adults with amoxicillin/clavulanate, 2nd or 3rd generation cephalosporin, or a quinolone. In the U.S., almost all are susceptible to erythromycin, tetracycline, and TMP/SMX.

Pseudomonas

Pseudomonas aeruginosa is a small Gram-negative rod with a single flagellum. Suspect *Pseudomonas aeruginosa* if there is a history of nail-puncture wounds (especially if through a tennis shoe), osteomyelitis and endocarditis in IV drug abusers, and acute or chronic otitis externa (which can be especially severe in diabetics). Ecthyma gangrenosum (round, indurated black lesion with central ulceration) accompanies pseudomonal bacteremia. *Pseudomonas* is the cause of "hot tub rash," which people get from improperly chlorinated hot tubs (this is usually self-limited).

Note

Enterobacteriaceae is a family of Gram-negative enteric bacilli and include: *Salmonella, Yersinia, Shigella, Citrobacter, E. coli, Klebsiella, Proteus, Serratia, Enterobacter,* and *Edwardsiella.* We'll discuss *Salmonella* and *Yersinia* now.

Salmonella

Salmonella are Gram-negative bacilli that are usually motile. Non-typhoidal *Salmonella* are a fairly common cause of diarrhea. Because the bacteria are not host-adapted like *S. typhi,* they can be found in many different, non-human host animals. It may be spread by frozen foods (especially chicken), milk, and eggs. Baby chicks, iguanas, turtles, and other exotic pets may also be sources of infections. Treatment increases the risk of developing a carrier state.

Salmonella typhi is, unlike most Salmonella, non-motile and encapsulated. It causes typhoid fever, usually from contaminated food, milk, or water. Adults are more likely to be carriers, because *S. typhi* tends to seed in gallstones (did "typhoid Mary" have gallstones?). The infection tends to cause leukopenia. The classic "rose spots" (See Image 2-11) form on the trunk about a week after the fever starts; these look like little, 2–3 mm diameter angiomas.

Recommend typhoid vaccine to travelers (> 2 years old) who go outside of the usual tourist areas of Latin America, Asia, and Africa. More on vaccination in the General Internal Medicine section.

Treatment of typhoid fever: Options include quinolones, 3rd generation cephalosporins, ampicillin, TMP/SMX, and chloramphenicol, depending on sensitivities. Carriers without gallbladder disease or stones can usually be cleared with 6 weeks of ampicillin + probenecid. (The probenecid decreases clearance and causes a higher blood level of the ampicillin.)

Yersinia

Yersinia pestis is a Gram-negative coccobacillus that causes plague. Reservoir is wild rodents. It is transmitted by fleas or direct contact (skinning animals) and has high mortality. The bubonic type causes large, localized lymphadenopathy ("buboes") that suppurates. If not treated, it can lead to sepsis and death. The bubonic type also may lead to a pneumonic form, which is rapidly transmitted to bystanders by coughing. (Bioterrorism has brought this organism back to the Board exam!) Note: Plague and tularemia present similarly (adenopathy after hunting, etc.), except that the geographic locations are different—desert S.W. for plague vs. Arkansas, Missouri, and Oklahoma for tularemia. More on tularemia below.

Diagnose plague by aspirating the lymph nodes.

Treat plague with streptomycin. 2nd line choices: tetracycline or quinolones.

Other *Enterobacteriaceae* are covered under "Diarrhea" in the Gastroenterology section.

Legionellaceae

The *Legionellaceae* family comprises many species—of which *Legionella pneumophila* causes 80–90% of human *Legionellaceae* infections. *Legionellaceae* are aerobic Gram-negative bacilli that require a particular medium to grow.

notes

Legionella is contained in water, and modes of transmission are multiple—with aspiration as the most likely.

Legionella pneumophila infection (legionellosis) causes legions of problems. Multisystem disease is the clue! Patients often present with diarrhea and CNS symptoms (H/A, delirium, and confusion), in addition to the pneumonia. Presentation is similar to, and often confused with, *Mycoplasma pneumoniae*. Like *M. pneumoniae*, the CXR is much worse looking than the exam indicates.

Treatment for moderate infections is azithromycin—or quinolones. If severely ill, add rifampin.

Klebsiella and other Gram-negative causes of pneumonia are covered in the Pulmonary section.

Brucella

Brucellosis is a zoonosis that is (worldwide) usually caused by *B. melitensis* (goats, sheep, and camels)—an aerobic Gram-negative bacillus. Other strains: *Brucella abortus* (cattle), *B. suis* (pigs), and *B. canis* (dogs). It is often transmitted to humans via unpasteurized milk or cheese or by inhalation (work-related). It affects the heart (especially suspect in culture-negative endocarditis), lungs, GI tract, GU (orchitis, abortion), and endocrine glands (thyroiditis, adrenal insufficiency, SIADH). Check for brucellosis in a FUO workup! Confirming the diagnosis is difficult. Cultures may take up to 6 weeks to grow. In some types, you can order serotyping (looking for increasing specific IgM titers).

Treatment requires combination therapy:
- doxycycline + aminoglycoside (streptomycin or gentamicin) x 4 wks, or
- doxycycline + rifampin x 4–8 wks.

Quinolones are effective for acute disease, but may have a higher relapse rate.

Francisella

Francisella tularensis is a small, Gram-negative pleomorphic bacillus that causes tularemia ("rabbit fever"). It is found in many animals. It is transmitted by ticks and blood-sucking flies, but the organism may also be ingested or inhaled. Especially seen in Arkansas, Missouri, and Oklahoma. Typically, patients with tularemia present with a history of sudden onset of fever, chills, myalgias, and arthralgias, followed by an irregular ulcer at the site of inoculation that may persist for months. Regional lymphadenopathy develops, and these nodes may necrose and suppurate.

Base the diagnosis of tularemia on the typical clinical presentation and confirm with serologic testing for *Francisella tularensis*. Differential includes plague, which occurs mostly in the desert S.W.

Treat with streptomycin, gentamicin, or tetracycline if not severely ill.

Bartonella

Bartonella bacilliformis causes bartonellosis, a disease that has 2 manifestations—severe/acute and chronic. *Bartonella* are tiny, Gram-negative pleomorphic bacteria. The disease is transmitted by sand flies only in the Andes Mountains (i.e., Peru). The only known reservoir is humans.

The initial, acute form consists of rapid onset of a febrile hemolytic anemia with a high mortality if untreated (50%)! This is called "Oroya fever." The chronic, benign form with chronic, cutaneous lesions is called "verruga peruana." *Salmonella* is a common cause of coinfection with Oroya fever. (Hmm! just as in the hemolytic anemia of sickle cell disease.)

Oroya fever usually responds dramatically to tetracycline or chloramphenicol. Chloramphenicol is preferred, because it also is effective against *Salmonella*.

Bartonella henselae causes cat-scratch disease (See Image 2-12) or, in the immunocompromised patient, bacillary angiomatosis. The skin lesions of bacillary angiomatosis are identical to "verruga per-uana" (above). Treatment: erythromycin +/- rifampin, depending on severity. Recent data support the use of azithromycin for treatment of cat-scratch disease. Note: Do not biopsy nodes.

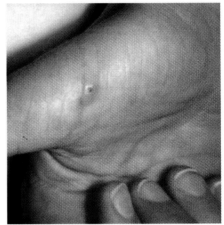
Image 2-12: Cat-scratch disease, 1° lesion

Helicobacter pylori

Helicobacter pylori is a Gram-negative, spiral, flagellated bacillus. It causes gastritis and PUD, and is a risk factor for adenocarcinoma of the stomach. *H. pylori* is discussed in the Gastroenterology section.

RICKETTSIAL

Rickettsia

Rickettsia rickettsii, a Gram-negative coccobacillus, causes Rocky Mountain spotted fever (RMSF)—[Know!] This disease has a 3% mortality. Classic signs and symptoms include a rash, fever, headache, arthralgias (but *not* overt arthritis), and a history of recent exposure to ticks. The rash occurs on the distal extremities (See Image 2-13). It progresses from maculopapular to petechial. Most infected persons get the rash, but few get all of the classic signs and symptoms. Patients may also present with diarrhea and abdominal pain.

notes

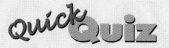
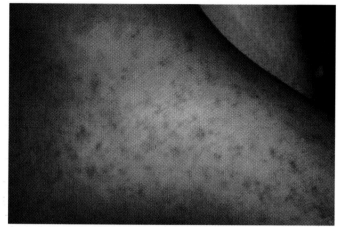

Image 2-13: Rocky Mountain spotted fever (RMSF)

Most clinicians diagnose this on clinical grounds, start treatment, and then confirm with serological testing. For a definite diagnosis, do immunofluorescent staining on a biopsy of the petechial lesion.

Other rickettsial infections include *R. typhi* (endemic typhus), *R. prowazekii* (epidemic typhus), *R. conorii* (Mediterranean spotted fever), and *Coxiella burnetii* (Q fever).

Know that Q fever is a zoonosis that is transmitted to humans mainly by inhalation of the aerosol released from the infected animal. Q fever is seen in abattoir (slaughterhouse) workers and people exposed to an infected animal's products of conception during birthing. Buzzwords: Cattle or Cats + Cilled (☹!) or Conception = Coxiella (Q fever).

Treat all *Rickettsia* infections with tetracycline/doxycycline or chloramphenicol. Quinolones are also effective. Vaccines have no effect.

Ehrlichia

Ehrlichia infection (ehrlichiosis) has been called "spotless Rocky Mountain Fever." Like RMSF, ticks are the transmission vector.

There are 2 forms of ehrlichiosis:
1) Human monocytic ehrlichiosis (HME)
2) Human granulocytic ehrlichiosis (HGE)

The organism is small, Gram-negative, and obligately intracellular. HME is due to *E. chaffeensis* and mainly seen in Missouri and Arkansas, while HGE is likely due to either *Anaplasma phagocytophila* (formerly *E. phagocytophila)* or *E. equi* and predominates in the NE and Upper Midwest U.S.

There is usually no rash. The organism affects the monocytes or neutrophils, and patients typically present with the viral picture of fever, headache, and leukopenia—they may also have thrombocytopenia. Think of this in a presentation of pancytopenia and tick bite!

Treatment is doxycycline/tetracycline.

Note: There are reports of dual infection with *Ehrlichia* + *Babesia microti* (an intra-RBC protozoan parasite) and *Ehrlichia* + *Borrelia burgdorferi* (Lyme) in the endemic Northeast areas.

GRAM-VARIABLE

Gardnerella vaginalis (previously called *Haemophilus vaginalis*) is Gram-variable. Treat with metronidazole. It is associated with a vaginosis. More on pg 2-46.

ACID-FAST

Mycobacteria

All *Mycobacteria* are acid-fast (red on a green background).

- *M. tuberculosis* can cause pleural effusions with a lymphocyte count of 1,000–6,000/mm^3, a low glucose, elevated protein, and elevated LDH. The glucose is normally > 80 although, in 20% of cases, it is < 60. More on TB in the Pulmonary section.

- *M. scrofulaceum* and *M. avium-intracellulare* cause lymphadenitis in children; treat by excising the nodes!

- *M. leprae* causes leprosy. Transmission is probably via respiratory droplets person-to-person. Diagnose with Fite stains of skin or nerve (See Image 2-14 and Image 2-15).

- *M. marinum* is the "fish-tank bacillus." It causes non-healing skin ulceration in people working around fish tanks. It often causes strings of lesions along the lymphatic channels. Treat *M. marinum* with ethambutol + rifampin or clarithromycin + rifampin (more on pg 2-47).

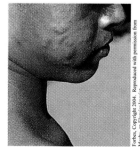

Image 2-14: Lepromatous leprosy

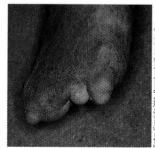

Image 2-15: Neurotrophic atrophy in lepromatous leprosy

Forbes, Copyright 2004. Reproduced with permission from Mosby, an Elsevier Imprint

notes

Nocardia

Nocardia asteroides is only weakly acid-fast (easily missed). Its shape is beaded, branching, and filamentous. It usually starts as a lung infection—occasionally causing a thin-walled cavitary lesion. It can cause focal brain abscesses and a neutrophilic chronic meningitis (most chronic meningitides are lymphocytic). Nodular skin lesions are common. It is hard to isolate.

Usual treatment is high-dose sulfonamides or TMP/SMX. In severely ill patients, add combinations of drugs including amikacin + imipenem. Minocycline is another alternate choice for those sulfa-allergic.

Nocardia brasiliensis is in the soil. Like *M. marinum*, it can cause inflammation with associated surface lesions along lymphatic channels. Treat with sulfonamides or TMP/SMX. Resistant to imipenem (But, *N. asteroides* is sensitive to imipenem).

Cryptosporidium and Isospora

Cryptosporidium and *Isospora belli* are both acid-fast, and both are common causes of chronic diarrhea in AIDS patients. The *Isospora* are large and oval-shaped; treat infection with TMP/SMX. Infection with *Cryptosporidia* (which are small and round) is usually self-limited in immunocompetent patients and requires no treatment; but for persistent diarrhea, nitazoxanide is now FDA-approved for immunocompetent patients. In immunocompromised patients, some have tried paromomycin and albendazole with varying success.

OTHER ORGANISMS

Actinomyces

Actinomyces is an anaerobic organism that causes an infection in which characteristic yellow "sulfur" granules grow, which are actually clusters of organisms. The usual presentation of actinomycosis is cervicofacial involvement caused by a dental infection (See Image 2-16 and Image 2-17). *Actinomyces* is a cause of PID when there is an IUD in place. Also, in the abdomen, be aware of *Actinomyces* associated with appendicitis. It occasionally causes a chronic, neutrophilic meningitis (as do *Nocardia* and fungi). Treatment is PCN or ampicillin. 2nd choice is tetracycline.

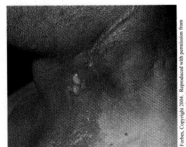

Image 2-16: Cervical actinomycosis

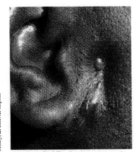

Image 2-17: Actinomycosis

Chlamydia / Chlamydophila

Chlamydia and *Chlamydophila* are obligate, intracellular parasites. *C. psittaci*, *C. trachomatis*, and *C. pneumoniae* (formerly TWAR) are pathogenic in humans.

- *C. psittaci* are found in psittacine and other birds and causes psittacosis: pneumonia and splenomegaly. Again: Any pneumonia associated with poultry, especially with splenomegaly, strongly suggests *C. psittaci* (DDx: *Histoplasma* also causes pneumonia and splenomegaly; it is associated with bird and bat droppings). Onset of psittacosis is associated with myalgias, rigors, headache, and high fever—to 105°F.
- *Chlamydophila pneumoniae* (TWAR) causes community-acquired pneumonia in adults who have not been exposed to birds; i.e., person-to-person spread. Bronchospasm is particularly prominent in respiratory infection caused by *C. pneumoniae*.
- *Chlamydia trachomatis* causes GU infections and trachoma (chronic, external eye infection causing cataracts, but not glaucoma; it is found especially in Asia and Africa). Approximately 5% of pregnant women have *C. trachomatis* in their genital tracts. The same *C. trachomatis* is also associated with neonatal pneumonia! Lymphogranuloma venereum is a STD caused by the same *C. trachomatis*, but a different immunotype.

ETC...

Sepsis is associated with an elevated WBC with left shift, increased PT and PTT, and metabolic acidosis; but overwhelming sepsis can cause leukopenia. Gram-negative septic shock is associated with warm extremities because, despite the decreased blood pressure, there is no compensatory peripheral vasoconstriction (i.e., peripheral vascular resistance numbers are low). Cardiac index is elevated (normal is 2.8–4.2 L/min/m^2).

Antibiotic prophylaxis is recommended for procedures associated with high risk of infection (such as hysterectomies, both vaginal and abdominal, and bowel surgeries), procedures involving implantation of prosthetic material (such as joint replacement), and some procedures when infections—if they occur—would be especially serious (cardiothoracic). The drug of choice almost always is cefazolin!

Staph, *Salmonella*, and *Serratia* are more likely to be seen in patients with granulomatous disease. And again: *H. influenzae*, *S. pneumoniae*, and meningococci are more likely in patients with spleen or antibody dysfunction. For dysfunctional T-cell–associated infections, see AIDS-associated infections on pg 2-36. *Aspergillus*, *Mucor*, and *Pseudomonas* infections are more likely in granulocytopenic patients (leukemia, chemotherapy, post transplant) than in AIDS patients.

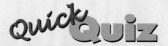
SPIROCHETES

SYPHILIS

Treponema pallidum causes syphilis. Sequence of infection:

- Primary syphilis presents with a painless chancre within 3–40 days (depending on the number of inoculating organisms) and regional lymphadenopathy. In women, if the infection is cervical, it is often asymptomatic. Chancre lasts 2–6 weeks, then resolves.

- Secondary syphilis occurs ~ 2 months later with generalized lymphadenopathy, constitutional symptoms, and mucosal (35%) and/or cutaneous (90%) lesions that can mimic many other lesions ("the great imitator"). The skin lesions may be macular or papular, but are rarely vesicular. They can occur on the palms and soles and are described as "nickels and dimes" lesions (See Image 2-18). These signs and symptoms resolve in 3–12 weeks, and the disease goes into a latency period. Untreated, 1/3 of secondary syphilis cases eventually proceed to tertiary syphilis.

- Tertiary syphilis: CNS lues (neurosyphilis; "lues" is just another word for syphilis), aortitis (aneurysm rupture is the main cause of death from syphilis!), and tabes dorsalis (causes demyelination, resulting in foot-slap and a wide-based gait). One CNS manifestation is the Argyll Robertson pupil, which is miotic (small) and irregular; it reacts normally to accommodation (contracts when focusing close, dilates when focusing on distant objects), but not to light.

Serology: There are 2 general types of tests:
1) Non-treponemal/reagin (VDRL and RPR) and
2) Treponemal (MHA-TP and FTA-ABS) tests.

20–30% of patients with primary syphilis are negative by either type of test, but will turn positive shortly thereafter. 99–100% of patients will be positive by either test in secondary syphilis. Once positive, the specific treponemal tests (MHA-TP and FTA-ABS) stay positive for life. The non-treponemal tests become negative after treatment unless treatment has been delayed for many years, in which case they may stay positive.

Scenarios [Know]:
1) −RPR, +MHA-TP:
   a) successfully treated for syphilis in the past, or
   b) early infection, or
   c) false-positive—see below. Check for history of Lyme disease and repeat RPR in 6 weeks.

2) +RPR, −MHA-TP:
   a) probably early infection, or
   b) often a false-positive in low-risk population. Repeat in 6 weeks.
3) +RPR, +MHA-TP: Infection

Antibodies to *Borrelia burgdorferi* (Lyme) cross-react and may cause a false-positive treponemal test (MHA-TP and FTA-ABS), but does not affect a non-treponemal test (VDRL and RPR).

If the VDRL or RPR becomes negative after treatment, it is a good indication of successful treatment. The non-treponemal tests may become negative in untreated persons with tertiary syphilis. So, secondary syphilis can typically be screened out by either test being negative; only the treponemal test can be used to screen out tertiary syphilis. I do not say "rule out" because, unfortunately, the false-negative rate in tertiary syphilis with the reagin (non-treponemal; VDRL and RPR) tests is up to 30%!

All pregnant women should get a non-treponemal test in the 1st trimester. If at high risk, repeat in the 3rd trimester and at delivery.

Note: All of the standard antibody tests in a newborn are positive if the mother was positive—because of crossover of IgG. The previously used newborn IgM test was not very sensitive, because the maternal IgG tended to "overwhelm" IgM response.

Note: More sensitive and specific newborn IgM tests check for *Toxoplasma*, rubella, and CMV.

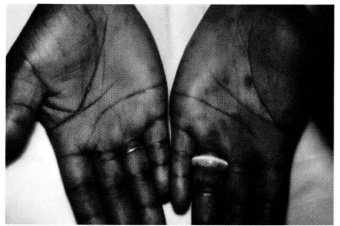

Image 2-18: Secondary Syphilis "nickles and dimes" lesions

notes

Treatment of syphilis:

For primary syphilis and for the early latency period of secondary syphilis (< 1 year since acquiring the disease):
- benzathine PCN G 2.4 MU IM or doxycycline 100 mg bid for 14 days.

Late latency secondary syphilis and tertiary syphilis with gummas or cardiovascular problems:
- benzathine PCN G 2.4 MU IM q week x 3 or doxycycline 100 mg PO bid x 4 weeks.

For neurosyphilis:
- PCN G 18–24 MU IV qd for 10–14 days. This is sometimes followed by benzathine PCN 2.4 MU IM q wk x 3. An alternative is procaine PCN 2.4 MU IM qd with probenecid 500 mg tid for 14 days. If PCN-allergic, the best course is to desensitize the patient according to CDC protocol, and give the PCN. Use ceftriaxone as an alternative for PCN-allergic patients with 2 grams a day for 10–14 days. Oral doxycycline is not effective for neurosyphilis.

Treat pregnant women and newborns for syphilis only with PCN. If the pregnant woman is PCN-allergic, desensitize her, then treat with PCN. After treatment, do a quantitative nontreponemal/reagin test monthly during pregnancy.

Procedures with newborns with possible syphilis:
- If the mother was ineffectively treated, not treated with PCN, treated < 4 weeks before delivery, or there is a clinical suspicion, treat the newborn with PCN.
- If treatment of the mother was sufficient, follow the infant's physical examination, CSF exam and nontreponemal serologic titers—and treat if there is a rise in titer or other abnormality.

Non-venereal treponemal diseases include yaws, pinta, and bejel.

LEPTOSPIROSIS

Leptospirosis is a spirochetal disease transferred by contact with infected animals or contaminated water. It is considered to be the most widespread zoonosis in the world. It causes a wide range of symptoms, from myalgias, fever, and headache with or without aseptic meningitis, to Weil's syndrome (severe hepatitis with renal failure and hemorrhagic complications—renal or hepatic symptoms may predominate). Pulmonary symptoms are also common. The hepatitis is characterized by the bilirubin being disproportionately elevated compared to the liver enzymes.

The variety of presenting symptoms makes for a high incidence of initial misdiagnosis. Clue: Look for contact with dog or rat urine.

Treat with PCN or doxycycline.

LYME DISEASE

Overview

Borrelia burgdorferi causes Lyme disease. It is transmitted by the *Ixodes scapularis* (previously *Ixodes dammini*) tick in the Northeast, and the *Ixodes pacificus* tick in the California area. (Remember that the protozoa *Babesia* is also transmitted by *Ixodes scapularis*—see pg 2-23.) Lyme disease can be found in virtually all of the lower 48 states. But (!), if you practice in Arkansas or Missouri, you will see ehrlichiosis more often than Lyme disease. The *I. scapularis* tick seems to be a better vector, so the disease is most prevalent in the Northeast, especially Martha's Vineyard and the Nantucket area. *Borrelia burgdorferi* does cross the placenta and causes fetal infection and death.

For the most part, ticks transmit Lyme disease during the nymph stage, probably because nymphs are more likely to feed on a person and are rarely noticed because of their small size (< 2 mm). Thus, the nymphs typically have ample time to feed and transmit the infection (ticks are most likely to transmit infection after ~ 2 or more days of feeding). If a patient says he had a tick on his body for 1 or 2 hours the previous day, just reassure him that no treatment is necessary.

Diagnosis of Lyme Disease

A definite diagnosis may be difficult to establish. Serology is negative in 90% of Stage I, so base the diagnosis on history plus clinical findings.

Stage I: Erythema migrans (EM) is the pathognomonic skin lesion of the early Stage I disease; it starts at the site of the bite, and is a slowly spreading, irregular erythematous lesion with a clear center (See Image 2-19).
Early symptoms include myalgias, arthralgias, fever, HA, and lymphadenopathy.

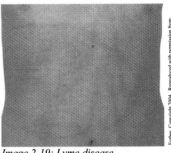

Forbes, Copyright 2004. Reproduced with permission from Mosby, an Elsevier Imprint

Image 2-19: Lyme disease

Then, weeks to months later, Stage II disease occurs with recurring erythema migrans (rare), neurologic problems (lymphocytic meningitis and/or neuritis), and heart problems (myocarditis, which may cause a rapidly alternating 1st, 2nd, or 3rd degree AV block). The neuritis often presents as a peripheral neuropathy, a cranial nerve palsy, or both; consider it in a patient with a suggestive history and Bell's palsy, foot-drop, or both.

Months-to-years later, Stage III occurs, most commonly, with arthritis (oligo- or migratory—small or large joints—usually large), but there can also be chronic neurologic syndromes.

Scenarios

Scenario 1: No prophylaxis is given for outdoor activities such as hiking and camping.

Scenario 2: If a patient presents with erythema migrans, do you want to check Lyme serology? The answer is no! Just Treat!

Scenario 3: if a patient presents with fatigue, joint stiffness (not arthritis), and muscle aches and/or tenderness, do you suspect Lyme disease? No! Do not check Lyme titers and do not treat for Lyme based on these non-specific findings!

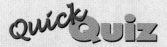
Scenario 4: For patients living in endemic areas who present with recurrent oligoarticular inflammatory arthritis, do an ELISA, followed by a Western blot; treat patients with positive results by either test.

Scenario 5: If same as scenario 4 but in a non-Lyme–endemic area, most authorities recommend treating only if both tests are positive.

Prevention and Treatment of Lyme Disease

There was a recombinant, outer-surface protein (OspA) Lyme disease vaccine (LYMErix®), but it was pulled from the market.

For the following treatments, keep in mind the the treatments are different for those with 1) early disease/Bell's palsy vs. 2) arthritis vs. 3) cardiac or neurologic disease [Know]:

1) Treat early disease and Bell's palsy with oral doxycycline or amoxicillin x 21 days.
2) Treat Lyme arthritis with oral agents, as above, then retreat with the same oral agent, or ceftriaxone if no response initially. Non-responders frequently are HLA-DR4 allele-positive.
3) Treat cardiac and neurologic sequelae with ceftriaxone 2 gms or PCN G 20 MU IV in divided doses x 21 days.

Other *Borrelia* infections are *B. recurrentis* and *B. vincentii*, which cause relapsing fever (in this, spirochetes are seen in the blood smears) and Vincent's angina, respectively.

OVERVIEW

Fungi are roughly divided into 2 morphologic types: yeasts and molds. There is also a dimorphic type that changes from a yeast to a mold, and vice versa, depending on temperature. The dimorphs are the type most likely to cause systemic disease in the immunocompetent host. The dimorphic fungi are also more limited in environment. The infecting form of fungi is usually spores (molds), which convert to yeasts in a moist environment at body temperature. The Deuteromycetes are a class of fungi containing the yeasts *Candida* and *Cryptococcus*, the molds that cause skin and nail disease (dermatophytes), and the dimorphic fungi: *Histoplasma*, *Coccidioides*, and *Blastomyces*. *Mucor* is of the class Phycomycetes (nonseptate hyphae), and *Aspergillus* is of the genus Ascomycetes.

CANDIDA

Consider *Candida albicans* as a cause of infection in immunosuppressed patients, patients on antibiotics (or doing poorly despite antibiotics), and patients with uncontrolled diabetes. Also consider it in patients with indwelling catheters. Diagnosis: On physical exam, determine disseminated candidiasis by finding a "cotton wool patch" on the retina. Swab all orifices and remove any catheters. Send the swabs and catheter tips for KOH and C+S.

Chronic, mucocutaneous candidiasis is associated with a T-cell problem, in which the T cell does not recognize *Candida*. It usually starts at an age < 2 years old. Patients present with a bad, chronic, oral and facial rash, alopecia, and occasionally, esophageal stricture. It is associated with polyglandular deficiency in which there can be hypoparathyroidism, Addison disease, DM, hypothyroidism, and/or vitiligo. These patients respond well to fluconazole. See pg 2-46 for *Candida* vaginitis.

Know: Candidemia can result in 3 deadly syndromes:
1) septic peripheral thrombophlebitis
2) septic thrombosis of the great central veins (especially with central venous catheters)
3) hepatosplenic candidiasis—consider this in recovering leukemia patients who present with fever and have negative cultures. CT scan shows focal areas of involvement of the liver.

Treat all of these by removing any infected catheter and giving appropriate antifungal therapy (see below). In addition, any suppurative peripheral vein must be resected. Suspect septic thrombosis of great central veins if there is edema of the upper body and/or candidemia persisting > 2 days after removal of the catheter.

Treatment: Even transient candidemia is now treated because of the increased possibility of secondary vertebral osteomyelitis, hepatic abscess, and endophthalmitis.

notes

For common *Candida albicans*, the following therapies can be used:

For non-neutropenic patients with candidemia, most recommend fluconazole 800 mg loading dose followed by 400 mg daily.

In stable neutropenic patients, fluconazole can be used unless they have received prior/recent fluconazole therapy.

For unstable neutropenic patients, an echinocandin is recommended. Amphotericin B is used much less frequently today because of the availability of these newer agents, which have much less toxicity.

CRYPTOCOCCUS

Cryptococcus usually causes minimally symptomatic, self-limited infections. Patients may have a low-grade fever, cough, and a pulmonary infiltrate—all of which resolve. It is not associated with any particular geographical location. Although it is found in old pigeon droppings, most patients have no recollection of being in contact with any. Cryptococcal pneumonia may form cavitary lesions and peripheral "cannon ball" skin lesions.

Dissemination is more likely in T-cell–deficient patients (AIDS, corticosteroid therapy, Hodgkin disease, ALL, diabetes, and those who are post-organ transplant). These patients are especially likely to get cryptococcal meningoencephalitis—the most common presentation of severe *Cryptococcus* infection.

Confirm presence of the organism with a CSF cryptococcal antigen test or a CSF India ink test, which is positive when you see the large "halo" due to the thick capsule around the organism.

Initially treat cryptococcal meningitis with amphotericin B and 5-fluorocytosine. Once the patient is clinically improved, these 2 agents can be stopped and the patient can be switched to fluconazole. Additionally, daily repeated lumbar punctures are recommended in those with increased intracranial pressure (> 200 mm H$_2$O) or with associated headache, clouded sensorium, visual/hearing loss, or cranial nerve palsies.

COCCIDIOIDES, HISTO, BLASTO

Note

Know all the following about coccidioidomycosis, histoplasmosis and blastomycosis!

Coccidioidomycosis

Coccidioides and *Histoplasma* are dimorphs, which are also discussed in the Pulmonology section. Neither usually causes much of a problem except in immunocompromised patients.

The spores of *Coccidioides immitis* are found in the soil of the arid southwest U.S. and northern Mexico (often called "Valley Fever"—think of San Joaquin Valley or Death Valley). Once inhaled, it converts to a yeast which, days to weeks later, causes a self-limited, flu-like illness with arthralgias, erythema multiforme, and/or erythema nodosum. It often has a sarcoid-like presentation. Disease often results in a pulmonary "coin lesion." In immunocompromised patients, the disease is usually more severe (see AIDS-related infections on pg 2-38). Think of this in a patient from Arizona with a sarcoid-like presentation!

Treat chronic coccidioidomycosis with fluconazole.

Histoplasmosis

Histoplasma is confined to the Mississippi and Ohio River valleys, and is especially found in bat and bird droppings. Do not confuse this with the "(Death) Valley fever" above.

Histoplasmosis can present with interstitial pneumonia, palate ulcers, and splenomegaly. 1/3 have anemia, neutropenia, or pancytopenia. The pneumonia and splenomegaly are similar to that seen in *C. psittaci* infection (pg 2-16). *Histoplasma* occasionally causes cavitary pneumonia similar to that seen in TB. Acute pulmonary disease generally requires no therapy. Chronic or severe, acute disease may be treated with itraconazole.

Treat disseminated disease with amphotericin B (either deoxycholate or liposomal formulations), followed by itraconazole.

Blastomycosis

Blastomyces causes blastomycosis, a flu-like illness similar to that caused by *Histo* and *Coccidio* above. It may also cause an acute illness that looks like bacterial pneumonia.

Blasto disseminates to the skin, usually causing verrucous (warty) lesions with central ulceration.

Bone lesions are common and may cause bone and joint pain.

Look for it in Arkansas and Wisconsin hunters and loggers.

Treat with itraconazole for mild to moderate disease and amphotericin B for CNS or severe disease

DERMATOPHYTES

Dermatophytes are the skin and hair fungi. Treat ringworm (*Tinea corporis*) with topical clotrimazole or undecylenic acid. Then, if no success, itraconazole or terbinafine are the preferred oral agents. Never amphotericin B.

SPOROTRICHOSIS

Sporotrichosis is caused by *Sporothrix schenckii*—a dimorphic fungus associated with plants. Gardeners tend to get it, often after being pricked by a thorn. Of the 4 types of clinical presentation, the cutaneous and the lymphangitic (nodules form on the skin over lymph channels) types are treated with oral potassium iodide or itraconazole, while the pulmonary and disseminated types are treated with itraconazole and, occasionally, amphotericin B. Sporotrichosis can be a chronic problem. The disseminated type is more common in immunodeficient gardeners! Warn those post-transplant rose gardeners! Remember: *Mycobacterium marinum* can cause similar lesions over lymphatic channels (see pg 2-47).

notes

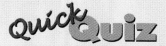

1) What type of fungal pneumonia can cause cavitary lesions and "cannon ball" skin lesions?

2) What test must you do on the CSF of a 1-month post-transplant patient with signs of meningitis?

3) Explain succinctly how to differentiate coccidioidomycosis, histoplasmosis, and blastomycosis. Based on geological region, and based on signs and symptoms.

4) What is the treatment for sporotrichosis?

5) What does the buzz phrase "diabetic with a black necrotic area in the paranasal sinuses" suggest?

6) What disease might you suspect in an AIDS patient with multiple mass lesions of the brain?

MUCORMYCOSIS

Mucormycosis can be caused by *Mucor*, *Rhizopus*, or *Cunninghamella* organisms. Pulmonary mucormycosis affects immunocompromised patients, causing pulmonary infarcts. In diabetics, sinusitis is more common. Rhinocerebral mucormycosis starts as a black necrotic spot in the nose or paranasal sinuses, and extends intracranially; it has a poor prognosis. Treat it with lipid amphotericin B and debridement. Posaconazole can be used as an option in those who cannot tolerate amphotericin B or for salvage therapy. Know that both *Aspergillus* and *Mucor* can cause a necrotizing, cavitating pneumonia.

PARASITES

PROTOZOA

Overview of Protozoa

There are 2 main types of parasites, Protozoa and Helminthic organisms. See Table 2-2.

The protozoa are single-celled and can replicate within the body, so it takes only a small number of organisms to cause infection. Protozoa do not cause eosinophilia.

The 3 types of protozoa are:

I. Sporozoa (*Toxoplasma*, *Cryptosporidia*, *Isospora*, *Pneumocystis* [although recent data support this more as a fungus!], *Plasmodium*, *Babesia*)

II. Ameba (*Entameba histolytica*)

III. Flagellates (*Giardia*, *Trichomonas*, *Trypanosoma*, *Leishmania*).

I. Sporozoa

Toxoplasma gondii

Toxoplasma gondii is the protozoan that causes toxoplasmosis. Cats are the definitive host since all the oocysts (infectious form) that eventually infect humans are shed in cat feces. It is common; 2/3 of adults have had it. Diagnose by finding an elevated IgM antibody. There are 4 types of toxoplasmosis:

1) In the immunocompetent, it is most often asymptomatic, but may cause nontender lymphadenopathy, night sweats, and atypical lymphs. Self-limited.

2) It is serious in the immunocompetent only if acquired during pregnancy, when it causes congenital toxoplasmosis (causing mental retardation and necrotizing chorioretinitis). The fetus is more likely to have a congenital infection if the disease is acquired later in pregnancy (15%: 1st trimester; 70%: last trimester, but those infected later in pregnancy are usually asymptomatic).

3) Immunocompromised patients tend to get CNS infection and multiple mass lesions caused by a reactivation of a latent infection. AIDS patients remain on therapy for life

Table 2-2: Classification of Parasites		
Group	Subgroup	Organism
PROTOZOA (DO replicate within the body) (no eosinophilia)	Sporozoa	*Toxoplasma, Cryptosporidium, Isospora belli, Plasmodium, Pneumocystis, Babesia*
	Ameba	*Entameba histolytica*
	Flagellates	*Giardia* - GI; *Trichomonas* - GU *Leishmania, Trypanosomes* - blood
HELMINTHS (do NOT replicate within the body) (+ eosinophilia)	Nemathelminthes (= nematodes) (= roundworms)	Pinworms, Hookworms, Whipworms (*Trichuris trichiura*), *Trichinella*, *Strongyloides*
	Platyhelminthes	Cestodes (tapeworms); Trematodes (flukes)

notes

unless immune reconstitution (normalized CD4 counts) has occurred with anti-retroviral therapy. Treat with pyrimethamine + sulfadiazine and leucovorin.

4) Ocular toxoplasmosis causes retinal lesions that look like yellow-white cotton patches, and also irregular scarring and pigmentation (disseminated candidiasis produces white cotton wool patches). Treatment consists of pyrimethamine and a sulfonamide (sulfadiazine or trisulfapyrimidine) for 3 weeks.

Cryptosporidium

Cryptosporidium is a protozoan that causes infection especially in the immunocompromised, but also in the immunocompetent. The oocytes are passed in animal (including human) feces (vs. just cats in toxo). Symptoms in immunocompetent patients usually consist of a watery diarrhea, which is self-limited, lasting 1–2 weeks. In the immunosuppressed, it can persist indefinitely and is refractory to medications—recent information shows that a combo of paromomycin + azithromycin may be helpful. Immunocompetent patients may be treated with nitazoxanide. Diagnose by acid-fast stains (small and round).

Isospora belli

Isospora belli is another acid-fast protozoan that causes a watery diarrhea in patients with AIDS, identical to *Cryptosporidium*. On the acid-fast stain, it is large and oval, whereas *Cryptosporidium* is small and round. Treat with TMP/SMX.

Cyclospora

Cyclospora is a newly described, acid-fast intestinal protozoan parasite causing diarrhea in immunocompromised and immunocompetent patients. Clue: **Raspberries** from Guatemala! Systemic symptoms such as malaise, myalgia, low-grade fever, and fatigue are commonly seen with *Cyclospora* infection. Treat with TMP/SMX.

Pneumocystis

Pneumocystis jiroveci ("yee-row-vet-zee"—previously termed *carinii*) is one of the most common causes of pneumonia in AIDS patients. It is covered later in this section in the HIV discussion and also in the Pulmonary section.

Malaria

Malaria—*Plasmodium* is a protozoan that causes malaria. It affects the RBCs and is transmitted via the *Anopheles* mosquito. There are 4 types: *P. vivax, P. ovale, P. malariae,* and *P. falciparum*. Asplenic patients have more severe cases of malaria.

P. falciparum is the worst type of malaria. It is the cause of virtually all of the fatal infections. It also has widespread chloroquine resistance. Most cases of *P. falciparum* are acquired in mid-Africa. The blood smear in *P. falciparum* shows "banana gametocytes," and often you see more than 1

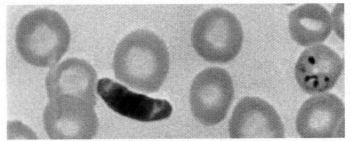
Image 2-20: P. falciparum, "banana gametocytes"

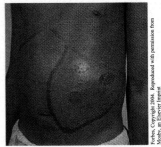
Image 2-21: Chronic malaria

infected RBC on the slide, and even multiple parasitized RBCs (See Image 2-20).

This greatly contrasts with the other forms of malaria in which the parasitized RBCs are often hard to find. Finding a banana gametocyte on the peripheral blood smear is diagnostic of *P. falciparum*. Even though *P. falciparum* causes the highest levels of parasitemia, the schizonts are not seen on peripheral smear. If you see schizonts, the patient has one of the other types.

The Duffy RBC antigen is the site of attachment for *P. vivax*. Any type of malaria can cause nephritis from immune complex deposition, but *P. malariae* is most commonly associated with nephrotic syndrome.

Antibody production causes a decrease in parasitemia, but not in the number of intracellular parasites!

Treatment (see Table 2-3): Use chloroquine for infections of *Plasmodium vivax, P. ovale,* and *P. malariae*. Primaquine is adjunctive medication for infections with *P. vivax* and *P. ovale* to eradicate hypnozoites in the liver (See Image 2-21). Hypnozoites are the malarial forms responsible for relapse. Treat chloroquine-sensitive *P. falciparum* with chloroquine, of course. If the *P. falciparum* is likely to be chloroquine-resistant, give quinine sulfate/gluconate, or others. Another option is mefloquine (Lariam®). Mefloquine is effective against chloroquine-resistant and even pyrimethamine/sulfadoxine-resistant *P. falciparum* (see next). It is also effective against the chloroquine-sensitive *Plasmodia*.

Remember: The use of pyrimethamine + sulfadoxine (Fansidar®) is rarely associated with the risk of severe Stevens-Johnson syndrome (which is due to the sulfa)! Also remember: Primaquine induces hemolytic anemia in G-6-PD–deficient persons, so you must screen for G-6-PD deficiency before prescribing it.

notes

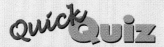

For malaria prophylaxis, use chloroquine if no chloroquine-resistant *falciparum* malaria is present in the area in question. Start it 1–2 weeks before patient departs to the endemic area and continue 4–6 weeks after she leaves the area. Use mefloquine or atovaquone + proguanil HCl (Malarone®), a fixed combination of atovaquone and proguanil HCl, for prophylaxis in chloroquine-resistant areas. Primaquine can be given the last 2 weeks of a prophylaxis period after travel to areas where there is *P. vivax* or *P. ovale*. Know that the main causes of malaria in the U.S. are either not taking prophylaxis or stopping prophylaxis too soon after returning from travel to endemic areas!

Atovaquone + proguanil HCl (Malarone®) is also approved for the prophylaxis and treatment of uncomplicated *P. falciparum* malaria. For prophylaxis, the advantage is that it can be started just prior to leaving, and stopped soon after return—and has fewer side effects. The disadvantage is that it must be taken daily.

Doxycycline has activity against chloroquine-resistant malaria, and can be used for prophylaxis at a dose of 100 mg daily. The advantage is that it is very inexpensive. The disadvantages are that it can cause photosensitivity, has to be taken daily, and has to be taken for 4 weeks after leaving the endemic area.

Babesia

Babesia microti is an intra-RBC protozoan parasite that causes babesiosis. This disease is a febrile, hemolytic anemia seen especially in debilitated elderly patients and asplenic patients. The organism is transmitted via the *Ixodes* tick from rodents (as is the spirochete *Borrelia*, which causes Lyme disease). It is most prevalent in the Northeast U.S.—usually in summer or early autumn.

Symptoms, which may persist for months, include fever, profuse sweats, myalgias, and shaking chills. Hemoglobinuria is a predominant sign. Patients often are emotionally labile. Because of the symptoms and the parasitized RBCs, it may be misdiagnosed as malaria.

B. microti is distinguished from *Plasmodium* by the classic intra-RBC pear shapes, which occasionally form a tetrad appearing as a "Maltese Cross" (See Image 2-22; the malarial parasites have a ring form).

Mild babesiosis infections are usually self-limited. Treat moderate infections with clindamycin + quinine or atovaquone + azithromycin. If severe, do an exchange transfusion, then give antibiotics. Asplenic patients have more severe disease. Again: Asplenic patients have more severe disease. And remember: Mixed infections with *Babesia*, *Ehrlichia*, and *Borrelia* are fairly common on the Boards.

Table 2-3: Prophylaxis and Treatment of Malaria		
Type of Malaria	**Treatment**	**Prophylaxis**
Nonfalciparum malaria	Chloroquine and primaquine	Chloroquine 500 mg (300 mg base) weekly. Give daily in endemic areas.
P. falciparum Chloroquine sensitive	Chloroquine Atovaquone + proguanil HCl	For all *P. falciparum*:
P. falciparum Chloroquine resistant Not very ill	Quinine sulfate PO plus either pyrimethamine + sulfadoxine, doxycycline, or clindamycin or Mefloquine 15-25 mg/kg; 1,250 mg max - single oral dose or Atovaquone + proguanil HCl: 4 PO qd daily x 3 days	Mefloquine: one dose weekly including 1 wk before and 4 wks after or
P. falciparum Chloroquine resistant Very ill	IV quinidine gluconate +/- IV clindamycin. When better, change to PO quinine and clindamycin	Malarone: one dose daily including 1-2 days before and 7 days after

notes

II. *Ameba*

Human amebiasis is caused by the protozoan *Entamoeba histolytica*. Transmission is fecal-oral and can be food- or waterborne. In the U.S., the usual population groups in which it is found are the institutionalized, immigrants, and homosexual men. For intestinal disease, diagnose by examining the stool.

However, the aspirate of an amebic liver abscess often shows no ameba or PMNs—Dx: serology!

Treat with metronidazole—even large amebic abscesses respond very quickly.

III. *Flagellates*

The flagellates: *Giardia lamblia*, *Trichomonas vaginalis*, *Trypanosoma*, *Leishmania*.

Giardia lamblia

Giardia infections are found in campers, travelers, children in daycare, homosexuals, and in patients with IgA deficiency and/or hypogammaglobulinemia. It infects the duodenum. (Remember: *Shigella* is also found among daycare kids and homosexuals). 75% of infected persons are asymptomatic. Acute symptoms include a watery, smelly diarrhea and flatulence. Chronic giardiasis causes flatulence, sulfuric belching, and soft stools. Diagnose with microscopic examination of fresh stool samples x 3 or *Giardia* antigen test on 1 stool. For chronic giardiasis, consider a string test—have the patient swallow a capsule on a string, leave it for several hours, then retrieve it and check for trophozoites. Note that this is rarely done today. Treat with metronidazole or quinacrine.

Trichomonas vaginalis

Trichomonas vaginalis causes an STD. Treat with metronidazole. More under Vaginitis, pg 2-46.

Trypanosomiasis

Trypanosoma causes trypanosomiasis. There are 2 main types. The African disease is sleeping sickness. It is caused by *Trypanosoma brucei* and is transmitted via the tsetse fly. The American illness, Chagas disease, is caused by *T. cruzi*; it is found in South America and Mexico. Usually, it is self-limited, but the chronic form can cause problems with the heart (from heart block to CHF), GI system (especially achalasia, megaesophagus, and megacolon, as discussed in GI section), and occasionally the CNS. Treat with antimonials and arsenicals obtained from the CDC. Note: Chagas disease is the most common cause of CHF in Brazil.

Leishmaniasis

Leishmaniasis is caused by any of the following 4 species of the *Leishmania* protozoa: *L. donovani*, *L. tropica*, *L. mexicana*, and *L. braziliensis*. *L. donovani* is spread by sand flies, and causes visceral leishmaniasis, also called kala-azar. These patients get GI symptoms, hepatomegaly, and sometimes huge splenomegaly. The other species cause cutaneous and mucocutaneous forms of the disease. Recent reports indicate there is a higher susceptibility for leishmaniasis in HIV-infected patients who travel to endemic areas.

Sodium stibogluconate (pentavalent antimony) is the treatment of choice—available from the CDC. Amphotericin B and itraconazole have been used with some success for cutaneous leishmaniasis.

HELMINTHIC ORGANISMS

Overview

The helminthic organisms are the other major type of parasite. (Remember: 1) Protozoa and 2) Helminthic organisms). Helminthic organisms are multicellular worms that, in general, do not replicate in the body—and they DO cause eosinophilia.

The 2 types of helminthic organisms are:
1) Nemathelminthes: the nematodes or roundworms that include pinworms, hookworms, whipworms (*Trichuris trichiura*), *Trichinella,* and *Strongyloides*, and
2) Platyhelminthes: include cestodes (tapeworms) and trematodes (flukes).

Nematodes (Roundworm)

Nematodes are the roundworms. We will mention 8 types:
1) Roundworm (*Ascaris lumbricoides*) (See Image 2-23).
2) Pinworm (*Enterobius*, causes rectal itching) (See Image 2-24).
3) Hookworm (e.g., *Necator americanus*, causes anemia, weakness and fatigue; also can cause cutaneous larva migrans) (See Image 2-25).

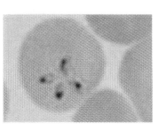

Image 2-22: Maltese Cross – Babesia microti

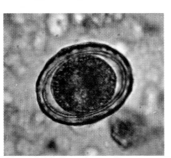

Image 2-23: Roundworm Egg

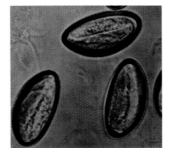

Image 2-24: Pinworm Eggs

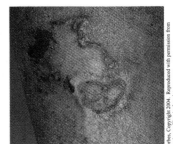

Image 2-25: Hookworm - Cutaneous larva migrans

Forbes, Copyright 2004. Reproduced with permission from Mosby, an Elsevier Imprint

notes

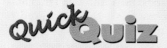

4) Whipworm (*Trichiura*).

5) *Trichinella spiralis* larvae, which are usually found in pork (but also in many carnivores), cause trichinosis. Although only ~ 50 cases per year are diagnosed in the U.S., the overall frequency of infection found on autopsy is ~ 4%! A recent U.S. outbreak occurred in Ohio due to bear meat from Canada.

6) *Wuchereria bancrofti* is transmitted by the mosquito. It is one of the causes of lymphatic filariasis (lymphatic blockage) and 2° elephantiasis! It may take thousands of bites by infected mosquitoes to inoculate enough of the organism to cause this (Remember: With the exception of *Strongyloides*, helminthic organisms do not multiply in the human body.) Diagnose by presence of microfilariae in the blood.

7) *Strongyloides stercoralis* is the least common of the nematodes in the U.S., but is very common in South America and Southeast Asia, where highly endemic areas have up to 60% of the population infected.

In the U.S., studies found infection rates of 3% among Kentucky schoolchildren and 6% at the Tennessee VA hospital.

It is (virtually) the only helminthic organism that replicates in the body. With this autoinfection, the infection can persist for decades (*Strong!*).

Symptoms are usually GI, but there can be pulmonary symptoms during the infective part of the larvae's life cycle.

Eosinophilia usually is present.

In immunosuppressed patients, potentially fatal disseminated strongyloidiasis may occur—presenting with abdominal pain and distension, neuro and pulmonary symptoms, and shock.

Diagnose with serial stool samples. Treat with ivermectin or thiabendazole.

8) *Toxocara canis* (and sometimes *Toxocara cati*) causes visceral larva migrans. The normal host for *Toxocara canis* is dogs, and it is transmitted to humans by ingesting soil contaminated with dog excreta. In humans, the larvae do not develop into adult worms but rather migrate through the host tissue—eliciting eosinophilia. In the U.S., *Toxocara* seropositivity is 20% in kindergarten children and 2% in the general population. Treat with albendazole or mebendazole.

Platyhelminthes (Cestodes and Trematodes)

Platyhelminthes include cestodes (tapeworms) and trematodes (flukes).

Cestodes are the flatworms (tapeworms). The pork tapeworm, *Taenia solium*, has 2 clinical entities:

1) If the cysticerci are ingested, taeniasis develops (a tapeworm grows in the intestines).
2) If an egg-contaminated food is ingested (from animal or human feces), the patient will develop cysticercosis. In this, the eggs hatch and the oncospheres go into the blood and, most significantly, cause cysticerci in the CNS and eyes. These cysts do nothing until the organism dies. In the brain (neurocysticercosis), the resulting inflammation usually causes seizures as the first symptom. Especially consider cysticercosis in a patient with new-onset seizures who is a Mexican immigrant, or from a household with a Mexican immigrant.

Niclosamide is the usual treatment for all intestinal tapeworms. Albendazole (1st choice) or praziquantel along with corticosteroids are used for neurocysticercosis. If ocular or spinal cysts are present, do not treat—this will cause irreparable damage.

Trematodes are the flukes.

1) *Clonorchis sinensis* is the Chinese liver fluke. It is endemic in the Far East; infection is caused by eating raw fish, and it is often associated with biliary obstruction.
2) *Schistosoma haematobium* infects the bladder, causing urinary symptoms.
3) *Schistosoma mansoni* is a fluke found in Africa, Middle East, and South America.
4) *Schistosoma japonicum* is found in Asia.

Schistosoma causes acute schistosomiasis (Katayama fever) ~ 2 months after inoculation. This infection presents with fever, lymphadenopathy, diarrhea (DDx: Travelers' diarrhea), hepatosplenomegaly, and marked eosinophilia. The most serious complication of schistosomiasis is cirrhosis with esophageal varices. Schistosomiasis does not cause the other stigmata seen with alcoholic cirrhosis (spiders, gynecomastia, or ascites) (See Image 2-26).

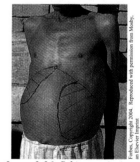

Image 2-26: Schistosomiasis with hepatosplenomegaly

Diagnosis: Finding the eggs in the stool or urine for *S. haematobium*.

Treatment: Praziquantel—give for one day!—for any *Schistosoma* and most other fluke infections.

notes

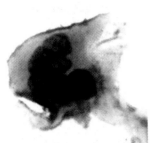

Image 2-27: Multinucleated giant cell

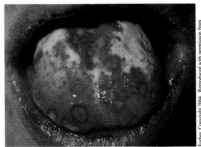

Image 2-28: Severe herpetic gingivo-stomatitis

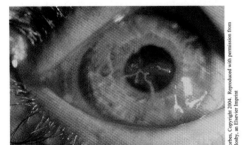

Image 2-29: A primary herpetic dendritic ulcer

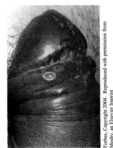

Image 2-30: Primary genital herpes

VIRUSES

HERPES SIMPLEX VIRUS (HSV)

Herpes Simplex Virus (HSV): A DNA virus.

HSV-1 causes orofacial infections in ~ 40% of the population. In the primary infection, the vesicular lesions and ulcers are usually localized to the oral mucosa, lips, and surrounding skin (See Image 2-28), whereas in recurrent infections, ulcers are usually on the outer lip.

Recurrent HSV-1 eye infection resulting in a keratitis is the most common infectious cause of blindness in industrialized nations (See Image 2-29).

Perform the Tzanck test by scraping down to the bottom cellular layer of a vesicle, placing the material on a slide, then staining with either Giemsa or Wright. In herpes simplex and varicella (including zoster), it will show multinucleated giant cells (See Image 2-27). Most centers no longer do the Tzanck test because it is neither sensitive nor specific; but be able to recognize the smear, because it commonly appears on Board exams. Viral culture, PCR, and DFA (next) have become the gold standards depending on the clinical situation. The use of HSV DFA (direct fluorescent antibody) test on lesions has become available in many centers. It is possible to autoinoculate the virus, so the infection can spread from the lips (or other areas) to the eyes of a patient.

HSV-2 causes "genital herpes." Actually, it causes about 75% of HSV genital infections—the rest are due to Type 1. Note that the prevalence of HSV-2 is 25% and of those, only 25% have symptoms! In 10% of patients, the initial occurrence of HSV-2 is associated with only a herpetic exudative pharyngi-

tis. New data suggest that many HSV infections are spread by asymptomatic shedding of virus.

Most cases of neonatal HSV are from intrapartum contact, so a C-section is recommended if the mother has symptoms or signs of genital herpes, or its prodrome, at the time of delivery. The risk for transmission to the neonate is high (30–50%) among women who get their 1st episode of genital herpes near the time of delivery and is low (< 1%) among women with a history of recurrent herpes. HSV reactivates in 2/3 of seropositive transplant patients within 6 weeks of transplant.

HSV causes the highest number of deaths due to encephalitis in adults (the most commonly identified etiologies are due to arboviruses, but the majority of encephalitis cases today are still not identified). Patients with herpes encephalitis usually present with constitutional symptoms and altered mental status, and may have focal neurologic signs. Because it has a predilection for the temporal lobe, patients may have temporal lobe seizure symptoms (abnormal behavior, smells burning rubber). > 60% will have neurologic sequelae! The EEG and MRI are the tests most sensitive for diagnosis. HSV PCR has also become more widely available, but is still less sensitive than MRI.

HSV is one of the many causes of erythema multiforme (See Dermatology section).

Treatment of HSV: Use acyclovir for all the types of herpes infections. Give IV in the immunosuppressed patients. Give it or one of its analogs (famciclovir, valacyclovir) orally for genital herpes. Acyclovir (or famciclovir, or valacyclovir) can also be given chronically to suppress infection, or as a treatment for acute recurrence. Use foscarnet to treat those with HSV resistant to acyclovir; ganciclovir is not used.

VARICELLA-ZOSTER VIRUS

Varicella-zoster virus (VZV; DNA) causes chickenpox (See Image 2-31) and herpes zoster (shingles). Symptoms of chickenpox are usually mild in children, but may be severe in adolescents and adults—especially pregnant women; pneumonia is more likely to occur in these older patients. In the pregnant mother, besides increased severity and pneumonia,

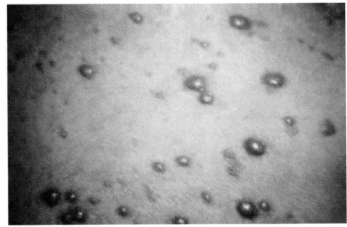

Image 2-31: VZV; Chickenpox

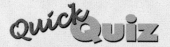

birth defects are more likely if she is infected between 8 and 20 weeks.

Current recommendation is for pregnant patients exposed to chickenpox to receive zoster immune globulin (VariZIG) within 4 days of exposure. If > 4 days, it does no good. Do not give varicella virus vaccine (Varivax®) to pregnant patients, because it is a live vaccine.

Most authorities recommend treating adults/adolescents with oral acyclovir 800 mg tid x 5 days if they present within the first 24 hours of the exanthem. Give IV acyclovir to immunocompromised patients.

Herpes zoster (shingles) is caused by reactivation of the varicella-zoster virus. A Tzanck smear shows multinucleated giant cells, which are pathognomonic for herpes viruses. Postherpetic neuralgia is more likely with increasing age. Shingles recurs in < 5% of non-immunosuppressed patients.

Prednisone, previously used with acyclovir, prolongs the course of herpes zoster in immunosuppressed patients. Immunosuppressed patients often get severe cases of shingles. Although it was previously thought that prednisone decreases the incidence of post-herpetic neuralgia in the immunocompetent, well-designed studies have shown no benefit.

Use high-dose oral acyclovir alone to treat zoster; although it shortens the course of acute illness a little, it does not decrease the incidence of post-herpetic neuralgia. Only famciclovir and valacyclovir are shown to decrease the incidence of post-herpetic neuralgia.

Valacyclovir is an L-valyl ester of acyclovir, has 3–5x greater bioavailability than acyclovir, and is almost completely converted to acyclovir after oral administration. For pain control, tricyclics, gabapentin, and lidocaine patches have some efficacy. Narcotics are effective and underused in this instance! Amitriptyline may be helpful for treatment of post-herpetic neuralgia.

If a patient presents with back pain and you think it is a herpes zoster prodrome, what should you do? Answer: Nothing, except follow closely. The acyclovir, or its analogs, is not started until you see the vesicles.

In 2006, the FDA approved and the ACIP recommended herpes zoster vaccination for all people aged 60 years and older. It is not recommended for pregnant women (hmm… > 60 and pregnant?) or those with primary or acquired immunodeficiencies. It is not recommended for the treatment of current zoster or postherpetic neuralgia.

CYTOMEGALOVIRUS (CMV)

Cytomegalovirus (CMV) is a DNA virus. CMV infection in the normal population is fairly common; 1/2 of the population has anti-CMV antibodies by the age of 35.

CMV infection in the normal population is usually asymptomatic but ~ 10% have a mononucleosis-type illness with fever, sore throat, adenopathy, fatigue, and hepatitis.

CMV is a very common infection in patients with decreased cellular immunity (post-transplant and AIDS). 75% of seronegative transplant recipients get CMV if the donor is seropositive. With a post-transplant systemic CMV infection, the patient can have concurrent "-itises," which may include encephalitis, hepatitis, retinitis, colitis, and adrenalitis (causing adrenal insufficiency); these are especially common and more severe if the recipient is seronegative prior to the transplant.

CMV is the usual cause of eye problems in AIDS patients with low CD4 count (especially < 200). CMV can cause chorioretinitis, pneumonitis, esophagitis, and colitis. The CMV retinitis is distinctive; it has both retinal blanching and hemorrhage. Confirm diagnosis with serum PCR for CMV DNA, which has replaced culture of the buffy coat smear as the test of choice. Diagnose CMV pneumonitis in transplant patients by finding inclusion bodies on the biopsy specimen.

Treat CMV chorioretinitis (usually in AIDS patients) with ganciclovir (DHPG), foscarnet, or a combination of both. Also, intraocular ganciclovir release devices with oral ganciclovir have been effective. Cidofovir is also approved. However, all of these agents have only a suppressive effect and must be given until T lymphocyte count increases to > 200.

Major toxicities of ganciclovir include granulocytopenia (30%!) and low platelets. ZDV (pg 2-32) also causes granulocytopenia, and patients occasionally cannot tolerate both. The major toxicity of foscarnet is reversible renal failure; it also causes hypocalcemia, hypomagnesemia, and hyperphosphatemia (patients may present with seizures). Because they are only suppressive, these drugs do not cure the symptoms; once they are stopped, the disease resumes.

EBV

Epstein-Barr Virus (DNA) causes infectious mononucleosis. Incubation period is 1–2 months. Most (> 90%) patients have pharyngitis or tonsillitis, fever, lymphadenopathy, and abnormal liver function.

EBV causes hairy leukoplakia; this mucocutaneous lesion may be seen as an early manifestation of HIV disease. Chronic fatigue has no proven association with EB virus.

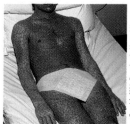

Image 2-32: Rash: infectious mononucleosis after using ampicillin

notes

The EBV is also associated with nasopharyngeal carcinoma and Burkitt lymphoma.

Recurrence is unusual but possible—usually with high titers of antibody to EB antigen (> 1:5000).

A patient with mononucleosis symptoms who is heterophil-negative usually has CMV.

Lymphocytosis is commonly found in EBV-infected patients with > 10% atypical lymphocytes: enlarged with abundant cytoplasm, vacuoles, and indentations of the cell membrane. 50% have splenomegaly. Most develop a macular rash if given ampicillin (See Image 2-32).

Heterophil antibody titers (monospot) decrease within 6 months, but the EB IgG antibodies are present for years. The atypical lymphs are T cells.

High-dose acyclovir may offer some benefit in treatment of oral hairy leukoplakia.

RUBELLA (GERMAN MEASLES)

Rubella is "German measles" (ss RNA virus) (See Image 2-33). If it is acquired by a pregnant patient in the 1st trimester, there is a 50% chance that the baby will have congenital defects. It is diagnosed by the hemagglutination inhibition test. If this test is negative in a newly exposed pregnant patient, repeat it in 3 weeks (after incubation period) before any decisions are made. If it is then positive, offer the patient the option of a therapeutic abortion. Immune globulin does not prevent the infection, but it may give some fetal protection in the patient who refuses therapeutic abortion.

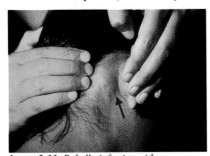
Image 2-33: Rubella infection with postauricular adenopathy

RUBEOLA (MEASLES)

Rubeola is "measles." Symptoms start ~ 10 days after the initial exposure. Symptoms at the onset: the "3 Cs": cough, coryza, and conjunctivitis (with photophobia). Patients also have malaise and fever. Koplik's spots (whitish spots on an erythematous base) appear on the buccal mucosa 2–3 days before the onset of the skin rash (See Image 2-34). The skin rash starts at the hairline and spreads downward. It lasts ~ 5 days and then resolves, also from the hairline downward. Again: 3 Cs, Koplik spots, rash. Outbreaks continue to occur, with the most recent occurring in Arizona and California in 2008.

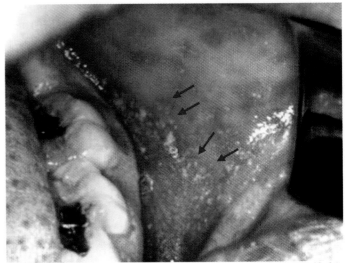
Image 2-34: Measles, Koplik spots. Small bluish-white spots that occur 12–24 hours before the rash.

RETROVIRUS

Retroviruses are RNA viruses.
- HTLV-1 causes T-cell leukemia and a neurologic syndrome, spastic tropical paraparesis seen in Japan and the Caribbean.
- HTLV-2 causes a rare T-cell variant of hairy cell leukemia.
- HIV, previously called HTLV-3, causes AIDS.
- HIV-2, found in W. Africa and parts of the U.S., is a virus that causes an illness indistinguishable from AIDS (both HIV I and II are now picked up by ELISA). More on HIV later.

RESPIRATORY VIRUSES

Rhinoviruses

Rhinoviruses are a common cause of URI in adults—usually during the autumn.

Respiratory Syncytial Virus

Respiratory syncytial virus (RSV) infections occur yearly, during the autumn and winter. RSV infections are more severe in the infant, occasionally resulting in pneumonia. Only 1% of affected infants are hospitalized. Diagnose RSV by doing an ELISA test on nasal secretions. Recent data show RSV to be as deadly as in influenza in the elderly, critically ill patient.

Influenza

Influenza is still a major cause of death, especially if the patient is > 55 years old with COPD. Vaccination decreases mortality by 1/3!

There are 3 types of influenza viruses: Influenza A, B, and C. A & B cause the yearly epidemics of respiratory illnesses. Influenza C causes very mild, if any, symptoms.

notes

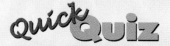

1) Which virus would you commonly see with atypical lymphocytes?

2) Which type of measles infection in a pregnant woman may cause consideration of a therapeutic abortion?

3) Which "spots" would you see in rubeola? What do they look like and when do they occur?

4) What drugs are used for Influenza A? Influenza B?

5) When is rabies preexposure prophylaxis indicated?

6) Always consider what 2 diagnoses in an adolescent who presents with enlarged parotid glands?

Treatment of influenza:

Oseltamivir (Tamiflu®—oral) and zanamivir (Relenza®—powder for inhalation) are the first of the neuraminidase inhibitors—a newer class of treatment for influenza A & B. If given within 48 hours of onset of symptoms, it decreases duration by 30%. If given within 12 hours, it decreases duration by 50%. It also prevents clinical disease in > 90% of household contacts. Today, these 2 drugs are the only effective agents. There was some hope that these agents would be successful against the "bird flu" strain (H5N1); however, resistance developed quickly!

Amantadine and rimantadine were previously used for influenza A. However, in the 2005-2006 influenza season, influenza A became resistant to these two antivirals, resulting in them being essentially ineffective.

What is the most effective way to prevent a nursing home outbreak of influenza? Answer: Immunize!

Know that starting in 2009, influenza vaccine will be recommended for all children from 6 months to 18 years (this includes adolescents—important for you to know this new group for the Boards!). Adults 50 and over and adults younger than 50 with chronic pulmonary, cardiovascular, renal, hepatic, and metabolic disorders, as well as those who are immunocompromised, should continue to be immunized as well.

The LAIV (live attenuated intranasal) vaccine may be used only in healthy individuals from 2–49 years of age. All others should receive the TIV (trivalent inactivated) injectable vaccine.

Coronavirus

Usual Coronavirus Infection

Coronavirus is an enveloped RNA virus. In its usual form, it is responsible for 3–5% of "common colds." It is more likely to be the etiology of the cold during the winter months.

Severe Acute Respiratory Syndrome (SARS)

Severe Acute Respiratory Syndrome (SARS) has now emerged as a concern, and is due to SARS-associated coronavirus (SARS-CoV). In 2003, there were > 8000 cases worldwide, and > 800 deaths. Be concerned about someone on the Board exam who presents with recent travel to Asia and who has early "flu-like" symptoms—but quickly progresses to severe respiratory distress. The elderly are more likely to be severely affected.

Vaccinations are covered in the General Internal Medicine section.

POLIO

90% of polio is self-limited. Its onset is characterized by an aseptic meningitis and an asymmetric, flaccid paralysis without reflexes. It is essentially eliminated in the western hemisphere and developed countries worldwide. More in the Neurology section.

RABIES

Rabies is especially found in bats, raccoons, skunks, and foxes. Not squirrels. If the animal is not available for rabies evaluation, and if the last vaccine was given > 6 years ago, give the vaccine and rabies immune globulin. Preexposure prophylaxis indicated for cave explorers and veterinarians, but not for hunters, mail carriers, etc. If suspect animals can be captured, a veterinarian should observe dogs, cats, and ferrets for 10 days for signs of rabies. Wild animals should be euthanized and tested for rabies, because observation in these animals is unreliable. On the exam, if a "bat is found in the room", then begin immediate rabies prophylaxis.

MUMPS

Mumps (RNA virus) occurs most commonly in winter and early spring. In 2006, a major outbreak occurred in Iowa and other states, making the virus more likely to appear on the Board exam. Although it often is asymptomatic, it can present with uni- or bilateral parotitis, aseptic meningitis, and/or encephalitis. 15–20% of post-pubertal males with mumps get an epididymo-orchitis, which is usually unilateral. Post-infection sterility is a rare occurrence. To differentiate mumps from bacterial parotitis, just check a Gram stain of the parotid secretions. There are many WBCs and organisms in bacterial parotitis and none in mumps.

Note: Another cause of enlarged parotid glands is frequent vomiting. Always consider bulimia in an adolescent or adult with parotid gland enlargement.

PARVOVIRUS

Parvovirus is a small DNA virus. One parvovirus, B19, causes various disorders, ranging from erythema infectiosum ("Fifth disease") to arthralgias/arthritis to aplastic anemia. Erythema infectiosum is a mildly contagious, self-limited infection that causes a rash and arthritis. The facial component of the rash causes a "slapped cheek" appearance. This rash is much

notes

more common in children, and the arthritis is more common in adults. It is in patients with chronic hemolytic anemias or AIDS that it can cause aplastic anemia. In these, the bone marrow shows characteristic "giant pronormoblasts."

ARBOVIRUSES

Arboviruses are mainly transmitted by mosquitoes or ticks. Various arboviruses occur in the U.S., typically in the late spring and summer. Until recently, most cases occurred along the Gulf Coast in Louisiana and Florida. Now, with West Nile virus, the arboviruses are seen from coast to coast. Today, West Nile virus is the most commonly identified arbovirus.

Besides West Nile, LaCrosse, St. Louis, Eastern Equine (EEE), Western Equine (WEE), Venezuelan Equine, Powassan, and Colorado tick fever viruses occur on occasion in the U.S. Almost all of these have similar symptoms: fever, headache, chills, and varied severity of encephalitis or aseptic meningitis. However, many cases are asymptomatic; only about 1/100 infected may present with symptoms.

Diagnosis: Finding virus-specific IgM antibody in the CSF or serum.

HANTAVIRUS

A hantavirus-associated disease, called Hantavirus Pulmonary Syndrome (HPS), starts with severe myalgias, fever, headache, and cough—and quickly progresses to ARDS and death. > 50% die. The primary reservoir in the U.S. is the deer mouse. On the Eastern coast and in the Southeast, the cotton rat is the main reservoir. The infection occurs when the excreta or saliva are inhaled. Transfer of the virus can also occur through the broken skin. No person-to-person transfer is known to have occurred.

Symptoms:
Early = constitutional symptoms in all. About 1/2 have N/V, diarrhea, and abdominal pain.
Late: 4–10 days later—coughing and shortness of breath as ARDS develops.
No rash. The clue: A young person with severe hemorrhagic pneumonia with decreased platelets and increased hematocrit.

DENGUE FEVER

Dengue fever, dengue hemorrhagic fever, and dengue shock syndrome are cause by any of 4 serotypes of the flavivirus. It is a tropical disease that uses humans and the day-biting *Aedes* mosquitoes (*Anopheles* carry malaria) in its life cycle. Dengue fever has had a resurgence during the last 10 years in South America and Mexico, with a few cases in South Texas. No vaccine is available yet (under development).

Symptoms: Rapid onset of high fever, severe myalgias, and arthralgias ("breakbone fever"), and severe headaches with N/V, followed by a macular red rash that covers most of the body. A second rash that looks more like measles occurs later, along with a recurrence of fever ("saddleback fever"—up, down, up).

Suspect this in a traveler with these symptoms who has returned from tropical latitudes (including the Caribbean and Mexico). Treatment is supportive.

SLOW VIRUSES

Overview

There are 2 classes of slow viruses.
1) normal viruses, such as papilloma (warts) and papovavirus (PML)
2) defective viruses, such as the defective measles virus, which causes subacute sclerosing panencephalitis

Papillomavirus

Papillomavirus causes warts. Genital warts are associated with an increased risk of cervical cancer. Many variants. HPV #1, 2, and 5 are common causes of plantar warts. HPV #6, 11, 16, 18, and 31 are genital. HPV # 6 and 11 are the cause of the exophytic, grossly visible genital warts, but only HPV #16, 18 and 31 are associated with cervical cancer (Remember: Higher numbers occur higher up on the body and are more cancer prone!). The HPV # 16, 18, and 31, which cause cervical cancer, are usually subclinical! So do not jump to "cervical cancer!" when you see genital warts! All warts tend to recur. HPV vaccine is now approved for females aged 9 to 26 years of age.

Papovavirus

Papovavirus—reactivation in the immunosuppressed host results in Progressive Multifocal Leukoencephalopathy (PML), which is due to progressive demyelination of the white matter. PML, because it is multifocal, has varied presentations. Usually, the patient suffers altered mental status, followed by various focal motor/sensory defects. Diagnosis: MRI.

Subacute Sclerosing Panencephalitis (SSPE)

Subacute sclerosing panencephalitis (SSPE) is a rare form of encephalopathy thought to be due to a measles virus that had been changed, but not eradicated, by the immune reaction to the primary infection. Occurrence is 1/300,000 cases of measles. Patients usually had measles at an age of < 2 years, and present with dementia, myoclonus, and new-onset seizures ~ age 10. Most die within several months of onset.

PRION DISEASE

Prions are proteinaceous infectious particles that lack nucleic acid and constitute a previously unknown means of transmitting disease. Previously, these diseases were thought to be caused by a "slow virus."

notes

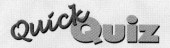

Quick Quiz

1) What virus presents as a rash in kids and arthritis in adults? How can this viral infection present in patients with AIDS?

2) What are the late symptoms of hantavirus infection. What are the early symptoms? What is the vector?

3) What viruses cause "breakbone fever"? In what group of patients, and with what symptoms, would you consider this diagnosis?

4) What types of genital warts are cancer-prone?

5) Which encephalitis is associated with early childhood measles?

6) Which prion disease is associated with progressive dementia and excessive startle response?

7) On the Boards, what diagnosis should you consider in a young adult from England who presents with worsening psychiatric problems and ataxia?

Prion diseases include Kuru, Creutzfeldt-Jakob disease (CJD), variant of CJD (vCJD), Gerstmann-Straussler-Scheinker (GSS) syndrome, and fatal familial insomnia. In animals, prions cause scrapie and mad cow disease (= bovine spongiform encephalopathy = vCJD when transmitted to humans).

Human prion diseases can be sporadic (CJD), infectious (vCJD, kuru, rare cases of CJD), or genetic (GSS syndrome, familial CJD, fatal familial insomnia).

Kuru is found in New Guinea, is associated with cannibalism, and is thought to be transmitted by ingestion of raw human brain tissue. It has an incubation period of up to 30 years. No new cases since ritual cannibalism stopped.

Creutzfeldt-Jakob disease (CJD) is the most common prion disease. It is almost always sporadic but ~ 5% are infectious (e.g., corneal transplants, cadaveric human growth hormone), and very few are genetic. Its incubation period is ~ 18 months. Patients with CJD get myoclonus and severe dementia. Neurologic symptoms predominate. They generally die within 5 months! There is no effective therapy for either kuru or CJD. The EEG is diagnostic.

A new variant of CJD (vCJD), probably transmitted from beef with bovine spongiform encephalopathy (mad cow disease), has been contracted by ~ 165 people worldwide, with most in the United Kingdom. No endemic U.S. human cases of vCJD have been reported. The only U.S. human cases so far were people who had moved from England. A case of bovine "mad cow" occurred in Washington State, traced to importation from Canada.

vCJD patients have early-on psychiatric symptoms and late-appearing neurologic symptoms (~ 6 months, ataxia). Once neurologic symptoms appear, progression to death is rapid. Boards: Look for a young adult from England with progressive psychiatric symptoms and ataxia.

HIV AND AIDS
OVERVIEW

Changes in the treatment and management of HIV infection are evolving rapidly. The following covers the basics—not the cutting edge. Recent Board examinations have steered clear of antiretroviral therapy, but they are still listed in the content specifications for the exams, so this information is presented here. However, realize that the Boards are more likely to focus on diagnosis and complications of disease than on having you start or change anti-HIV medications.

The virus particle:

The HIV virus is composed of a dense, single-strand RNA core surrounded by a lipoprotein envelope. The RNA contains reverse transcriptase, which allows the RNA to be transcribed into DNA, which is then assimilated into the host's genome. The cell then becomes an HIV-producing machine.

The structure in the lipoprotein envelope that allows the HIV to attach to the CD4 cell is named gp120. As opposed to influenza, the envelope on HIV is very unstable and, therefore, it is much more difficult to make a vaccine against it.

HIV gp120 envelope glycoprotein binds to the CD4 receptors and coreceptors on the helper T cells, macrophages, and monocytes. The virus fuses with the cell, and the viral core material enters the cell. Immune dysfunction results from the ongoing destruction of CD4 lymphocytes (this will be more fully described under "Summary of Important Advances"). The CD4 cells are the major regulator cells in the body. They can suppress the B lymphocytes, and regulate the CD8/suppressor cells.

With the decrease in CD4+ counts, B cells become deregulated and are no longer suppressed, causing a polyclonal increase in total serum immunoglobulins, even though overall antibody function is decreased! For this reason, infectious diseases in AIDS patients not only include the cell-mediated infections (PCP, viruses, *Mycobacteria*, and fungi), but also those seen with humoral deficiency (pneumococcus, meningococcus, *H. influenzae*, and *Giardia*).

The glial cells of the CNS may be directly affected by HIV, causing atrophy and dementia. The GI epithelium may be directly infected, causing a wasting enteropathy with diarrhea. Marrow progenitor cell infection may be the cause of anemia and thrombocytopenia.

Prevalence and transmission: HIV is positive among 50% of IV drug users and 50% of gays seeking treatment for STDs. Prevalence is < 1% in heterosexuals in the U.S., but in central Africa, heterosexual transmission is the primary route!

Associations in AIDS patients in the U.S.: homosexuals (56%), IV drug users (24%), IV drug user & homosexual (5%), heterosexual contact (6%), hemophiliacs (1%), transfusion-associated (2%).

HIV infection is diagnosed by demonstrating the presence of the virus or antibody to the virus.

Antibody is detected by means of the ELISA test, which is 99% sensitive and 90% specific. Positive responders are confirmed by the Western blot. Antibody to HIV is usually detectable 2–3 months after inoculation, although there can be a window of up to 6 months!

The earliest detectable sign of infection is a positive HIV PCR DNA, and this can be positive within a few days of inoculation. This HIV PCR DNA test is a positive/negative test that determines if HIV is there at all.

The usual method of determining viral load, once infection is confirmed, is with one of several tests that measure the actual levels of HIV RNA by amplifying the RNA—by oligonucleotide hybridization or enzymatic methods (can be PCR). An important question was recently answered: The level of HIV RNA (viral load) achieved by antiretroviral therapy has the same predictive value as that in untreated patients.

Again:

1) ELISA test for HIV antibody is the usual means of determining HIV infection. A positive test is confirmed by Western Blot.

2) HIV PCR DNA test is a qualitative (yes/no) test used to determine if there is HIV infection, and it is typically used only to determine if there is early infection. Once positive, it stays positive.

3) HIV PCR RNA test, and others like it, determines actual RNA levels, which may be undetectable in a person under treatment for HIV infection.

TREATMENT OF HIV INFECTION

Note

Treatment of HIV infection: Adherence is a key determinant in the degree and duration of viral suppression! AIDS: Note that it is extremely important to actively involve the patient in the treatment decision-making process. Guide decisions regarding initiation or changes in antiretroviral therapy by monitoring plasma HIV RNA (viral load) and CD4 T cell counts, in addition to the patient's clinical condition.

First, we will review the 6 major classes of anti-HIV drugs, then the treatment protocols.

Drug acronyms for the 6 major classes (color-coded to decrease probability of gutless crying):

1) NRTI = Nucleoside Reverse Transcriptase Inhibitor
2) Nucleotide RTI = Nucleotide Reverse Transcriptase Inhibitor
3) NNRTI = Non-Nucleoside Reverse Transcriptase Inhibitor
4) PI = Protease Inhibitors
5) FI = Entry/Fusion Inhibitors
6) Integrase inhibitors

Nucleoside Reverse Transcriptase Inhibitors

Nucleoside Reverse Transcriptase Inhibitors (NRTIs): These drugs inhibit the replication of HIV by interfering with the reverse transcriptase enzyme. These are all analogs of normally occurring nucleic acid bases.

Zidovudine (ZDV) = Azidothymidine (previously called AZT) = Retrovir®. This is the oldest of the antiretroviral drugs, but still remains very useful. It is well tolerated at currently used doses, but causes bone marrow suppression (anemia, granulocytopenia) and myopathy. A macrocytosis (elevated MCV) always occurs, but has no clinical consequence. ZDV does not usually cause problems for the kidneys or lungs, and does not cause pancreatitis.

As with all antiretroviral drugs, combination therapy is preferred and is the standard of care. ZDV is used in combination with 3TC, ddI, as well as protease inhibitors. Do not use ZDV and d4T together due to antagonism. The effectiveness of all drugs decreases over time if they are used in regimens that are not fully suppressive.

Give ZDV to HIV+ pregnant patients, because ZDV decreases transmission of the HIV virus to the fetus by 25–35%!

Because ganciclovir and ZDV have overlapping bone marrow toxicities, in an AIDS patient with CMV retinitis and on ZDV and ganciclovir, filgrastim (Neupogen®; G-CSF) can be given to support the WBCs. Sometimes, it is necessary to stop the ganciclovir and use foscarnet.

ddI (didanosine, Videx®) is useful in combination regimens—with ZDV, d4T (less commonly used with ddI due to increased toxicity and should be used only if no other agent is available), and protease inhibitors. Viral resistance develops more slowly than with other reverse transcriptase inhibitors. A newer, enteric-coated tablet has replaced the regular preparation with elimination of the GI side effects of diarrhea and cramping and, hence, much better patient tolerance.

The most severe side effects are pancreatitis, which can be life-threatening, and peripheral neuropathy. There is no bone marrow toxicity. Fatal lactic acidosis can occur with concomitant use of d4T.

d4T (stavudine, Zerit®) has emerged as a very useful drug because it is very well tolerated over long periods of time with little toxicity. Well-studied combinations include d4T/3TC with or without protease inhibitors. Recent data have implicated d4T in lipodystrophy and mitochondrial toxicity syndromes. Also, d4T should not be used in combination with ddI in pregnant women—fatal lactic acidosis!

Side effects: especially pancreatitis and peripheral neuropathy.

3TC (lamivudine, Epivir®) is a very effective drug in combination therapy. Combinations with ZDV or d4T are often used. The drug is well tolerated. 3TC is the most commonly prescribed antiretroviral agent.

Side effects are rare.

FTC (emtricitabine, Emtriva®, Coviracil®) is a drug that is extremely effective in combination therapy. It has minimal tox-

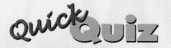

icity. FTC is an analog of 3TC and exhibits complete cross-resistance.

Abacavir (Ziagen®) is very effective in combination therapy.
Side effects: The most serious reaction is a hypersensitivity reaction, which usually occurs within 4 weeks. The reaction consists of a generalized rash and/or a flu-like illness with fever, chills, N/V, myalgias, cough, and shortness of breath. Remove abacavir from any patient who develops this reaction and never give it again; re-challenge causes an accelerated hypersensitivity reaction that causes multiple organ failure and can be rapidly fatal.
Abacavir hypersensitivity is linked to the HLA type B-5701 gene, and now it is recommended that all patients be tested for this gene before beginning abacavir therapy. If negative, the hypersensitivity rate decreases to < 2%.

Combos: Currently, there are 5 combination NRTI drug formulations:
• Combivir® (ZDV + 3TC)
• Trizivir® (ZDV + 3TC + abacavir)
• Epzicom® (abacavir + 3TC)
• Truvada® (FTC + tenofovir)
• Atripla® (efavirenz + FTC + tenofovir).
Trizivir can be used as single therapy because it contains 3 NRTIs, but it is viewed best as an alternative therapy since long-term outcomes are poorer with Trizivir alone.

Nucleotide Reverse Transcriptase Inhibitor

Tenofovir (Viread™) is a nucleotide-RTI very similar to the above nucleoside analogs, except that nucleotide-RTIs are chemically pre-activated and, therefore, require less biochemical processing than the nucleoside RTIs.

Tenofovir has once-daily dosing and a good side-effect profile—mainly asthenia/headache/N/V/D/flatulence. Azotemia has been seen with tenofovir, particularly in patients predisposed to renal disease. Tenofovir must be taken *with* a NRTI *and* at least 1 PI or NNRTI. Avoid the combination of tenofovir and ddI because of drug interactions and intracellular accumulation of metabolites that can actually cause T lymphocyte levels to drop.

Non-nucleoside Reverse Transcriptase Inhibitors

Nevirapine (Viramune®) is the first of this class of drugs. It is not useful as a single agent, but is useful as part of a regimen with nucleoside reverse transcriptase inhibitors and/or protease inhibitors. Rash, which can be severe, is the primary toxicity. Fatal hepatic toxicity, especially in women with higher CD4 counts and patients coinfected with hepatitis, has been reported.

Efavirenz (Sustiva®) is more potent than nevirapine. CNS toxicity is commonly seen. Efavirenz is teratogenic, and is absolutely contraindicated in pregnancy and discouraged from use in women of child bearing potential. Other side effects include rash and "weird dreams."

Etravirine (Intelence®, Celsentri®) was approved in 2008. Monitor for serious skin rash. It is useful in HIV-infection that has been previously resistant to the other NNRTIs. Delavirdine (Rescriptor®) is less potent and, therefore, rarely used.

Protease Inhibitors

HIV protease inhibitors—PI (saquinavir, indinavir, ritonavir, nelfinavir, lopinavir, fosamprenavir, atazanavir, tipranavir, and darunavir) inhibit the HIV protease enzyme that is involved with processing the completed virus. They must be used either in combination with other PIs (e.g., saquinavir + ritonavir), or with the just discussed NRTIs +/– NNRTI to prevent the emergence of resistance. Fat redistribution and lipid abnormalities (increased triglycerides and cholesterol), as well as new-onset diabetes, have been recognized with the use of PIs. However, in treating the lipid abnormalities, do not use simvastatin or lovastatin with any of the PIs! Also avoid other drugs that cause interactions: Rifampin, astemizole, cisapride, and St. John's wort.

Saquinavir (Fortovase®) is highly effective, has minimum side effects, and is useful in combination protease inhibitor regimens.

Ritonavir (Norvir®) is a very potent drug, but patient tolerability is poor due to side effects. The main side effects are N/V, flushing, distorted taste, and paresthesias. There are many drug interactions because of interference with the p450 enzyme system. Low-dose ritonavir inhibits metabolism of, and significantly boosts, levels of indinavir, saquinavir, fosamprenavir, lopinavir, tipranavir, darunavir, and atazanavir. Ritonavir is now usually used in low doses to boost the levels

notes

of other PIs and used with efavirenz, since efavirenz tends to lower levels of some PIs.

Indinavir (Crixivan®) has side effects that include an asymptomatic hyperbilirubinemia and a high incidence of nephrolithiasis. The drug should be taken on an empty stomach with adequate hydration—although boosting with ritonavir eliminates the food requirement. Indinavir is rarely used because of the development of PIs that are less toxic and have more convenient dosing.

Nelfinavir (Viracept®) is a PI with good potency. Most common side effect is diarrhea. If resistance to nelfinavir develops, treatment with other agents may be effective. Recently, nelfinavir was recalled for use in pregnancy because of conatminants in the preparation. It is less commonly used because of the GI intolerance and the better efficacy of the newer PIs. Nelfinavir is the only PI that cannot be boosted with ritonavir, and hence its activity cannot be enhanced.

Fosamprenavir (Lexiva®) is the prodrug of amprenavir, a PI no longer available. It requires fewer pills and eliminates the major side effects of amprenavir.

Lopinavir/ritonavir (Kaletra®) is a co-formulation of lopinavir and low-dose ritonavir. Lopinavir is available only in this co-formulation. It is very potent and well tolerated. Most consider Kaletra the "gold standard" of PIs.

Atazanavir (Reyataz®) is a once-daily PI that doesn't have adverse lipid effects. For maximum potency, the drug needs to be boosted with ritonavir.

Tipranavir (Aptivus®) was approved in late 2005. It has adverse lipid effects, and its main side effects are GI-related and rash. It is limited to highly resistant virus.

Darunavir (Prezista®) was approved in 2006. Monitor closely in patients with underlying hepatitis coinfection. It has maintained activity against highly resistant virus.

Entry/Fusion Inhibitors

Enfuvirtide (Fuzeon®) is the only fusion inhibitor available. Give by subcutaneous injection. Its main side effects are local reactions at the injection site and increased risk of bacterial pneumonia. It is not part of most regimens.

Maraviroc (Selzentry®) is the first drug approved for treatment of CCR5-tropic HIV. It blocks HIV from entering human cells. It is an oral agent.

Integrase Inhibitors

Raltegravir (Isentress®) is the only integrase inhibitor currently available. It prevents the HIV integrase enzyme from inserting HIV's genetic information into an infected cell's own DNA, halting this critical step in the life cycle of HIV. It is an oral agent.

Key Words

Key word/phrases to remember for side effects:
- ZDV: bone marrow suppression and myopathy
- The "D's" (ddI and d4T): pancreatitis and peripheral neuropathy
- Abacavir (Ziagen®): potentially fatal hypersensitivity reaction
- Efavirenz (Sustiva®): teratogenic; CNS side effects (bad dreams)
- Indinavir (Crixivan®): kidney stones

Note about all the medications above: At least know the yellow-highlighted areas!

State of Treatment
Summary of Important Advances

1) HIV RNA assays are available for accurately determining viral load. Prior to the availability of these assays, most believed the HIV virus entered a prolonged latency period until the onset of symptoms. It turns out that there is continuous, high-level replication from the onset of infection to death.

2) Viral load is a good, long-term predictor of outcome. After primary infection, the rate of virus replication and turnover equilibrates to a certain set point for each individual—resulting in a pretty much constant plasma viremia of 100-to-10^6 HIV RNA copies/mL. This set point may endure for months or years, and it determines the rate of disease progression. Plasma viremia < 5,000 HIV RNA copies/mL is associated with near-normal CD4+ counts and minimal if any clinical progression of disease, whereas viral loads > 30,000 HIV RNA copies/mL indicate a greatly increased risk of disease progression. Barring treatment, a single HIV RNA count can establish a prognosis—similar to staging of certain malignancies.

Infected patients make up to 10^9 new HIV virions/day. The CD4+ lymphocytes, which are the principal cells targeted for reproducing HIV virions, have a half-life of only 1.6 days after infection. High levels of viremia cause tremendous and continuous CD4+ lymphocyte destruction—eventually causing decreased levels. Rather than using CD4+ cell level as a marker of disease activity (which is wrong—it is more an endpoint denoting prolonged disease activity), the present focus of treatment is to decrease viral load and, thereby, prevent or minimize the CD4+ cell destruction. And, as mentioned before, it is now known that the viral load achieved by antiretroviral therapy has the same predictive value as that in untreated patients.

3) The HIV protease inhibitors decrease viral load—sometimes tremendously—for prolonged periods when used in combination therapy.

4) Always use combination therapy for HIV. Treat with PI(s) or NNRTI in combination with NRTI for initial therapy. Combinations of nucleoside analogs given to asymptomatic pa-

notes

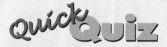
tients with early HIV disease, and evidence of immunologic compromise (low CD4 counts), prolong survival and decrease AIDS-related problems. The combination therapy is superior to ZDV alone. Previously, no one knew if early treatment in the course of the illness would improve outcome.

Pending Questions

1) How long-lasting is the effect of the protease inhibitor agents? HIV does mutate but the lower the viral load, the less the likelihood of resistance developing, and the longer the regimen will be effective. Patients have been maintained without detectable virus for > 12 years.
2) What is the best combination of agents? Guidelines are becoming less vague and more proscriptive (see below).
3) When is the best time to start treatment? Some guidelines (see below), but still vague for asymptomatic patients.

The New Treatment Protocols are Based on the Above and:

1) The finding that the decrease in viral load induced by combinations or ART (anti-retroviral therapy) have good predictive value.
2) Determining CD4 and viral load are key indicators for when to start therapy.
3) Combination therapy is the standard of care—use monotherapy only in special circumstances.

Indications for Viral Load Testing

1) Syndrome consistent with acute HIV
2) Initial evaluation of newly diagnosed HIV
3) Every 3–4 months for patients on and not on therapy
4) 2–8 weeks after initiation of therapy
5) Clinical event or substantial decline in CD4 count

Indications for Using Drug-Resistance Assays

Resistance testing is now a standard of care. They are indicated for naïve patients before initiating treatment and whenever treatment is changed because of viral resistance. Currently, 2 types of resistance testing are available—genotypic and phe-

notypic. The genotypic test will detect specific genes in the individual patient's HIV virus known to confer resistance toward a specific antiretroviral drug. The phenotypic test determines if the gene is operating and if resistance is being expressed. For patients with pretreatment HIV RNA > 1000 copies/mL, genotypic resistance testing is recommended. Genotypic testing is recommended over pheyotypic testing in the treatment naïve patient. Either or both concurrently can be used in the setting of increased viral load with presumed HIV-resistance to help determine change in therapy. This is sort of like a crude antibiogram for the HIV virus—if resistance is determined, then you can switch from ineffective drugs.

When to Initiate Antiretroviral Therapy

Definite:
- Symptomatic (AIDS or severe symptoms): start therapy no matter what the CD4 or viral load
- Asymptomatic and CD4 is < 350
- Pregnant women
- Persons with HIV-associated nephropathy
- Persons coinfected with hepatitis B

Some recommend:
- Asymptomatic with CD4 > 350 and viral load is ≥ 100,000 copies/mL.

Also, know that a finger stick from an infected needle requires immediate treatment with 3-drug antiretroviral therapy.

Be aware: The optimal time to initiate therapy is unknown among persons with asymptomatic disease with CD4 count > 350. Base all decisions regarding the start of therapy on prognosis, as determined by CD4 and viral load and the willingness of the patient to adhere to therapy.

Which Combination of Drugs to Use

Treatment regimens are now either "NNRTI-Based" or "PI-Based:"

NNRTI-Based—**preferred:**
- Efavirenz + abacavir/lamivudine (remember to test for HLAB*5701!) or
- Efavirenz + tenofovir/emtricitabine

Remember not to use efavirenz in the 1st trimester of pregnancy or in women who are likely to become pregnant. Note that as of April 2008, controversy exists regarding use of abacavir and the increase risk of myocardial infarction. As of this time, DHHS was monitoring the situation, but did not recommend a change in the current recommendations.

NNRTI-Based—alternative:
- Nevirapine + ZDV/lamivudine or
- Nevirapine + ddI + (emtricitabine or lamivudine)

Use with caution in those with high CD4 counts (women > 250, men > 400), because of increased hepatic events (11% in women with CD4 > 250!) with nevirapine.

notes

PI-Based—preferred:
- Start with atazanavir or fosamprenavir or lopinavir
- and add ritonavir to one of the above
- and add either abacavir/lamivudine or tenofovir/emtricitabine.

PI-Based—alternative:
- 10 different combinations—Unnecessary for you to know for the IM Board exam

When to Change HIV Therapy:

This again is controversial. However, 2 things to know:
1) Don't change drugs based on 1 viral load; always repeat a high viral load to be sure it is not lab error.
2) Intolerance to the medication should prompt evaluation for change of therapy.

Reasons to change therapy on treatment failure (various definitions and not standardized):
- Therapy has not suppressed viral RNA to undetectable levels (< 50 copies) within 4–6 months of starting therapy.
- An increase of ≥ three-fold from the nadir of plasma HIV RNA.
- Previously undetectable levels now surpass 1000 copies.

The other problem is what drug to change to? Generally, just know you should probably change therapy based on resistance testing.

Post-Exposure Prophylaxis (PEP)

First, determine the exposure risk: Was the source material blood or bloody fluid? If so, then determine if it was a percutaneous exposure (yes—PEP recommended), or mucous membrane or skin with compromised integrity (PEP probably recommended). It is easier (and frequently asked on tests) to remember whom not to give PEP to: Do not give for intact skin exposures and urine-source exposures. The current thought is to use potent combination therapy. Treatment should start ASAP—within hours of exposure. The standard regimen is ZDV, 3TC, +/- lopinavir/ritonavir for 4 weeks.

Pregnancy and HIV Drugs

Treat all pregnant HIV-infected women with ART regardless of CD4 level. The goal is to make her viral load undetectable.

If she is already on ART and it is suppressing viremia, continue her current regimen except avoid use of efavirenz. If she is not on ART at time of pregnancy, initiate therapy based on antiretroviral drug resistance testing and include ZDV if feasible. Do not use nevirapine as a component if her CD4 count is > 250.

All pregnant women should be given ZDV as a continuous infusion during labor in addition to their current ART therapy.

Schedule Cesarean delivery at 38 weeks gestation if plasma HIV RNA remains > 1000 copies near the time of delivery.

Infants born to HIV-infected mothers should receive ZDV for 6 weeks starting within 6–12 hours of birth.

Suppressing the viral load in the mother lowers the risk of transmission to the newborn. The bottom line for most pregnant women: Treat with ART, include ZDV if possible, and do not use efavirenz (teratogenic) or a D4T/ddI combination (increased risk of lactic acidosis in pregnant women). C-section is now recommended if viral load cannot be suppressed below 1000 copies.

HIV-ASSOCIATED INFECTIONS AND CONDITIONS

Introduction

Signs of HIV disease include persistent or recurrent seborrheic dermatitis, *Taenia* infections, psoriasis, molluscum contagiosum, folliculitis, and mucocutaneous infections (hairy leukoplakia, herpes, oral or vaginal candidiasis). [Know these.] Hairy leukoplakia is caused by EBV.

Kaposi lesions are a neoplasia of blood vessels and are due to human herpesvirus 8. Lesions are heaped up and well localized, often with some surrounding bruising.

Don't forget the Acute Retroviral Syndrome: This is a flu or mononucleosis-like syndrome that occurs 2–4 weeks after initial infection and lasts 1–2 weeks. Patients present with fever, lymphadenopathy, pharyngitis, rash (usually erythematous maculopapular with lesions on face, trunk or extremities, including palms and soles), mucocutaneous ulcerations involving the mouth, esophagus or genitals, and myalgias/arthralgias. Consider it in a young person who has multiple sexual partners/IV drug user, and presents with signs/symptoms of mono or scarlet fever.

You can do a coronary artery bypass (CABG) on an HIV patient if he or she has a > 10-year prognosis.

PCP and HIV

Pneumocystis jiroveci (formerly *P. carinii*) pneumonia (PCP) is the most common opportunistic infection in AIDS patients. It is the presenting illness in 50% of AIDS patients. It is probably the most common lung infection overall in these patients but, because prophylaxis is so effective, PCP incidence in AIDS patients is decreasing to less than that of *S. pneumoniae* in some places.

Presentation of PCP: insidious onset of fever, shortness of breath, and dry cough.

Lab: ABGs show a pH > 7.40. A-a gradient is wide. Hypoxia is common. PCO_2 is low (from respiratory alkalosis). LDH is elevated (> 400), and liver enzymes are normal. The chest x-ray usually shows a diffuse "batwing" infiltrate, although it may also be lobar or unilateral. Occasionally, the chest x-ray is normal.

Again: PCP usually has an insidious onset; if an AIDS patient presents with an acute onset of pulmonary symptoms, first get a sputum for Gram stain and C+S, and start empirical treatment for community-acquired pneumonia.

notes

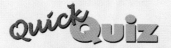
Patients who are most susceptible for PCP have a CD4 count < 200, so all of these patients should receive PCP prophylaxis.

The best method of diagnosis is by methenamine silver stain of samples taken by bronchoscopy or BAL, although induced sputum is effective in up to 50% in some hospitals. CMV is usually grown along with PCP from BAL/bronchoscopy samples; only rarely is this significant.

Treat mild PCP with oral TMP/SMX, or atovaquone if unable to tolerate TMP/SMX.

Treat more severe PCP—P_aO_2 < 70 or A-a gradient > 35—with PO or IV TMP/SMX or IV pentamidine and high-dose corticosteroids (start on the first day). Inhaled pentamidine is not recommended for treatment of PCP. If there is no response after 1 week, or if severe side effects develop, switch. Alternative treatments are dapsone + trimethoprim, clindamycin + primaquine, or atovaquone alone for mild-to-moderate cases. PCP patients must receive 21 days of effective therapy. Remember: Include steroids for any patient with a P_aO_2 < 70!

Side effects: Both TMP/SMX and pentamidine can cause neutropenia/leukopenia. TMP/SMX side effects include skin rash, nausea/vomiting, and occasionally fever. Pentamidine causes fever, nausea, vomiting, and diarrhea. Pentamidine also causes azotemia and renal failure. Recurrent courses of pentamidine destroy the islet cells of the pancreas, causing hypoglycemia, which may not be reversible. (If a patient treated with pentamidine seizes, check fingerstick glucometer!) Hyperglycemia may also occur with pentamidine. Patients on aerosolized pentamidine are at risk for apical pneumothorax. For some patients with AIDS, the reactions to either TMP/SMX or pentamidine are intolerable, and you must change the medication.

Prophylaxis of PCP: Again, start when CD4 count < 200. Give TMP/SMX DS (or SS) once daily or one DS 3 times weekly. If patient cannot tolerate, give dapsone or atovaquone.

Atovaquone is more efficacious than dapsone and has a lower incidence of side effects than TMP/SMX but is much more expensive than either. ~ 4% of patients on TMP/SMX discontinue therapy because of rash.

• TMP/SMX is more effective.
• TMP/SMX gets extrapulmonary *Pneumocystis jiroveci*, whereas aerosolized pentamidine does not.
• TMP/SMX also prophylaxes against toxoplasmosis.

Stopping primary PCP prophylaxis (i.e., no history of these infections):
If CD4 > 200 for ≥ 3 months in response to ART (antiretroviral therapy), discontinue PCP prophylaxis. Remember that PCP prophylaxis is started when CD4 < 200.

Stopping secondary PCP prophylaxis (+ history of these infections):
If CD4 > 200 for ≥ 3 months in response to ART, discontinue PCP prophylaxis.

Mycobacterium and HIV

Tuberculosis is also common in AIDS patients, sometimes without infiltrates, and hardly ever with cavitation. Patients usually respond very well to treatment. Do a TB skin test on all persons who are seropositive for HIV. Treat a positive PPD (> 5 mm) without sign of disease with INH for 9 months. Treatment of active TB in a patient with AIDS is the same as in regular patients. See Pulmonology section for treatment.

M. avium Complex (MAC, *M. avium-intracellulare*) is a common, usually disseminated infection in patients with AIDS. It causes a wasting syndrome with fever, weight loss, and night sweats. There is no cure. Clarithromycin or azithromycin, in combination with ethambutol and sometimes other agents, including rifabutin, quinolones, clofazimine, or amikacin, can be beneficial in decreasing fever or improving bone-marrow function.

Today, a main therapy is treatment of the underlying HIV, allowing reconstitution of T-cell function.

Start primary prophylaxis for MAC with clarithromycin or azithromycin when CD4 < 50.

Stop primary prophylaxis (i.e., no history of these infections) when CD4 > 100 for ≥ 3 months in response to ART.

Stopping secondary prophylaxis (+ history of these infections):
MAC: Controversial on if and when you can stop MAC prophylaxis with a history of MAC. Most would stop if CD4 > 100 for 3 months.

Pulmonary: Other

Cryptococcus also involves the lung and can be disseminated, but it also commonly goes to the CNS. Cryptococcal meningitis is strongly associated with AIDS, Hodgkin disease, ALL, diabetes, and those who are post-organ transplant.

Treat with amphotericin B +/- flucytosine, *then* follow up with oral fluconazole. Always include flucytosine in AIDS patients!

Be careful! Flucytosine (5-FC; 5-fluorocytosine) rarely causes bone marrow suppression.

Histoplasma can either affect the lung or disseminate in AIDS patients (only non-AIDS patients have the calcified lung lesions). It can affect many organ systems, including the bone marrow. Think of this when an HIV-positive patient presents with interstitial pneumonia, palate ulcers, splenomegaly, and bone marrow suppression. This infection is very common in natives of El Salvador. Treat with itraconazole or amphotericin B. See pg 2-20.

Coccidioides: Again lungs, but it also can disseminate. It is associated with arthralgias, arthritis, hilar adenopathy, erythema multiforme, and erythema nodosum (similar to sarcoidosis). Treatment suppresses, but usually does not cure, this disease, so chronic suppressive treatment is needed (usually daily fluconazole—1st choice—or amphotericin B).

Know: Both *Aspergillus* (especially associated with marijuana use) and *Mucor* can cause a necrotizing, cavitating pneumonia in AIDS patients.

Pseudomonas infections are more prevalent in granulocytopenic patients (leukemia, chemotherapy, and post-transplant) than in AIDS patients.

GI and HIV

If AIDS patient has esophagitis, think of *Candida*. Not all *Candida* esophagitis is associated with thrush. If the patient does not respond to treatment for *Candida*, consider CMV esophagitis.

Chronic diarrhea in AIDS patients is usually caused by *Cryptosporidium*, *Salmonella*, *Shigella*, *Cyclospora*, or *Isospora belli*. *Cryptosporidium* shows up as small, round, red organisms ("round bodies") against a green background on acid-fast staining of the specimen. There is no reliable treatment of cryptosporidiosis. Nitazoxanide is the preferred drug. *Cyclospora* and *Isospora belli* are also acid-fast (*I. belli* is large and oval); treat both with TMP/SMX.

Neuro and HIV

Subacute diffuse encephalitis (caused directly by HIV) is a common neurologic problem in patients with AIDS.

Toxoplasma gondii is the most common cause of "AIDS-associated, enhancing-focal-space-occupying-lesions" (but the differential diagnosis also includes CNS lymphomas). CT scan shows CNS abscesses due to *Toxo* as ring-enhancing lesions. They are usually multiple but may be single.

If you see ring-enhancing brain lesions in any AIDS patient, start empiric treatment for CNS toxoplasmosis:
long-term pyrimethamine + a sulfonamide (usually sulfadiazine) or clindamycin (if sulfa allergic) + folinic acid.

Syphilis, even if previously treated, may reactivate in AIDS patients and cause neurosyphilis!

Any eye problems are probably due to CMV retinitis (see pg 2-27).

Summary: Stopping PCP or MAC Prophylaxis

Stopping primary prophylaxis (i.e., no history of these infections):

PCP: If CD4 > 200 for ≥ 3 months in response to ART (antiretroviral therapy), discontinue PCP prophylaxis. Remember that PCP prophylaxis is started when CD4 < 200.

MAC: If CD4 > 100 for ≥ 3 months in response to ART, discontinue MAC prophylaxis.

Stopping secondary prophylaxis (+ history of these infections):

PCP: If CD4 > 200 for ≥ 3 months in response to ART, discontinue PCP prophylaxis.

MAC: Controversial on if and when you can stop MAC prophylaxis with a history of MAC. Most would stop if CD4 > 100 for 3 months.

COMMON ID SYNDROMES

HEART: BACTERIAL ENDOCARDITIS

Introduction

Bacterial Endocarditis—See Cardiology section for prophylaxis indications and medications. See Table 2-4 (in this ID section) for treatment and diagnosis. Blood cultures are vital in diagnosing endocarditis of any type and should be drawn before empiric antibiotics are started. Blood cultures are usually positive (95%!) due to the constant level of bacteremia. If they are negative (and patient has not been partially treated with antibiotics), think of fungi, Q fever (*Coxiella burnetii*), *Legionella*, *Chlamydia psittaci*, nutritionally deficient streptococci, and the HACEK organisms (discussed below) as possible causes. Surgery is required for endocarditis with fistula, abscess, pericarditis, or persistent fever, and for cases in which the resulting valve dysfunction causes ventricular failure. In the heart, the electrical conduction pathway passes just beside the aortic valve; a conduction disturbance in a patient with aortic valve endocarditis is another indication for surgery. Vegetations alone usually are not an indication for surgery.

Again: CHF with endocarditis is an indication for cardiac surgery, and mortality in endocarditis surgery correlates with the pre-op severity of ventricular failure. The most common cause of cardiac death due to endocarditis is congestive heart failure.

ABE vs. SBE

There are 2 methods of classification of endocarditis. The classic method is based on acuity of presentation: acute vs. subacute. The more recent method is based on pertinent etiologic factors: native valve, prosthetic valve, addict (i.e., IV drugs), and culture-negative. These may have acute or

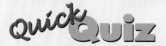

1) Which fungal disease do you think of in AIDS patients presenting with palate ulcers, splenomegaly, and neutropenia?

2) Which valvular lesion is most commonly associated with native valve endocarditis?

3) What are Janeway lesions?

subacute presentations. Addict and culture-negative can also be thought of as subsets of native valve and prosthetic valve endocarditis. In Table 2-4, they are shown only as subsets of native valve, because this is the setting in which they generally occur. The distinction is important because the frequency of occurrence of the various organisms is different in each group.

In acute, native valve endocarditis, *S. aureus* is the most common cause (40%). Next in frequency is pneumococcus, and then Group A streptococcus. All of the streptococcal infections = 35%. The following occur with ~ 5% frequency each: enterococci, Gram-negative organisms, and *S. epidermidis*.

Overall (acute and subacute), the major organisms are *S. aureus* and viridans group streptococci.

In addicts, the major organism is, again, *S. aureus* (50%), followed by enterococci (15%). The following 3 have a frequency of 7–8% in this group: *Strep*, Gram-negative (usually *Pseudomonas* or *Serratia)*, and *Candida*.

In prosthetic valve endocarditis occurring up to 1 year after surgery, by far the most common organism is *S. epidermidis* (55–60%).

ABE

Acute bacterial endocarditis (ABE) is caused by virulent bacteria, often attacking normal valves. It has an acute course in which there is often rapid cardiac valve destruction and resultant ventricular decompensation. There is ~ 50% mortality with *Staph aureus* endocarditis despite early intervention! The only common peripheral manifestations of ABE are Janeway lesions, which are small, nontender macules on the palms and soles. With *Staph*, sometimes peripheral ecchymoses appear. Embolization (again, especially with *S. aureus*) of the heart vegetations leads to metastatic infection (especially to the CNS and kidneys).

Table 2-4: Bacterial Endocarditis – Diagnosis and Treatment – Native vs Prosthetic Valve

Classification	Subsets	Presentation	Initial approach	Empiric treatment while awaiting C&S results	Culture results	Normal treatment based on organisms per C&S
Native valve	Non-addict	Acute	*A	1. PCN/amp + naf/ox or cefazolin + gent	*S. aureus* (40%)	(Naf/ox or cefazolin) +/- gent
					S. pneumoniae	PCN G/amp + gentamicin
		Subacute	*S	1. Same as #1 above OR 2. Get C&S results before antibiotic therapy	*S. viridans, S. bovis* (colon cancer!), other strep, *Enterococcus*	PCN G/amp +/- gentamicin; check for PCN and gentamicin resistance with *Enterococcus*
	Addict	Acute	*A	Same as #1 above	*S. aureus* (50%); *Pseudomonas;* Other Gram-neg bacilli (*Serratia marcescens, Enterobacteriacea*)	*S. aureus:* same as for non-addict. *Pseudomonas:* same as for *S. aureus*
		Subacute	*S	Same as #1 or #2 above	*Enterococcus* (15%) *S. viridans* Fungal	*Enterococcus:* Amp + gent; check for beta-lactam and gent resistance Fungal: amphotericin B + 5-FC
	Culture neg, Non-addict	Subacute	*S	Same as #1 or #2 above	HACEK organisms (50%)	Amp + gent or ceftriaxone
					Fungal, also consider Q fever (*Coxiella burnetii*), *C. psittaci*	Fungal: amphotericin B
Prosthetic valve	Early postsurgery (< 2 mo)	Acute	*A	Vanc + gent + rifampin	*S. epidermidis* (55-60%)	Vanc + gent + rifampin for 14 days then vanc + rifampin for 4 weeks
					S. aureus, Strep, cult neg (each <10%)	*S. aureus:* (Naf/ox or cefazolin) +/- gent
	Late postsurgery (> 2 mo)	Subacute	*S	Vanc + gent + rifampin	*S. epidermidis* (55-60%) *S. viridans* *S. aureus*	Vanc + gent + rifampin for 14 days then vanc + rifampin for 4 weeks

*A: Draw 1st set of BC and start empiric tx. Note: Acute presentation often includes Janeway lesions.
*S: Draw 3-4 sets of blood cultures over 24 hours and then initiate empiric treatment (some physicians elect to wait for results with subacute presentation.). Note: Subacute presentation, if caught late, may include Osler nodes and Roth spots. Note: SBE suggests a preexisting valvular abnormality. The above antibiotics give you a general feel for the treatment, but there are many other equally valid treatments.
Note: If PCN allergic, give ceftriaxone or vancomycin for PCN-sensitive; vancomycin for PCN-resistant; Vanc + gent for *Enterococcus*; vanc for *S. aureus*.

notes

SBE

Subacute bacterial endocarditis (SBE) usually occurs in patients with underlying cardiac disease.

KNOW these manifestations: low-grade fever, heart murmurs, conjunctival petechiae, splenomegaly (in 2/3), splinter hemorrhages, Roth spots, and Osler nodes. Patients may have fever and weight loss, and anemia and thrombocytopenia.

Roth spots are pale retinal lesions surrounded by hemorrhage. Osler nodes (= OUCHlers nodes) are ~ 0.5 cm tender nodules found on the palms, fingertips, and soles. Roth spots and Osler nodes are late developments of SBE and are seen less frequently today because of earlier diagnosis and treatment of SBE. Remember: you find Janeway lesions (nontender macules) in ABE, usually not SBE.

Native Valve Endocarditis

Native valve SBE is more common on the left side of the heart, and usually occurs on regurgitant AV valves (although it can also occur with VSDs and PDAs). Mitral valve prolapse is the most common valve lesion associated with native valve SBE! Prosthetic valve endocarditis is seen even more often. *Strep viridans* (from the oropharynx) is the most common cause of SBE, then enterococcal group D *Strep* (GI, urinary tract), then non-enterococcal group D *Strep*. In SBE, embolization of the heart vegetations only rarely leads to metastatic infection.

Strep bovis, one of the group D streptococci, is the only type that is easily killed by PCN alone. The other non-enterococcal group D *Strep* requires an aminoglycoside + a beta-lactam antibiotic (2 'cidal antibiotics). *S. bovis* endocarditis is associated with colon cancer.

Enterococcus requires ampicillin and gentamicin (not streptomycin). This is why the empiric treatment for endocarditis usually includes naf/ox (for *Staph*) + PCN (required for *Enterococcus*) + gentamicin (for all).

There are some cases of fastidious, Gram-negative organisms causing SBE. They are called the "HACEK" organisms (*Haemophilus*, *Actinobacillus*, *Cardiobacterium*, *Eikenella*, and *Kingella*), and usually are sensitive to beta-lactams. In culture-negative endocarditis, it was previously thought one of the HACEK organisms would be likely: *Haemophilus*, *Actinobacillus*, *Cardiobacterium*, *Eikenella*, and *Kingella*. However in the modern microbiologic era, fastidious organisms (zoonotic agents and fungi) and streptococcal species, especially in those who have received previous antibiotic therapy, are the most common causes of culture-negative endocarditis. (A prospective study showed *Coxiella burnetii* was found in 48%, *Bartonella* in 28%). Treat HACEK infection with PCN + gentamicin or ceftriaxone or per culture results.

Question: If you see Roth spots or Osler nodes in a patient, what is the treatment? Answer: In SBE, draw 3–4 sets of blood cultures over 24 hours before starting antibiotics. Some elect to wait for the C & S results before initiating SBE treatment.

Also remember: Endocarditis caused by either *Strep bovis* bacteremia or *Clostridium septicum* sepsis is directly tied to colon cancer in 10–25% of cases, so conduct a thorough GI check in these patients.

Prosthetic Valve Endocarditis

Prosthetic valve endocarditis (PVE) can be acute or subacute in presentation.

Early PVE (< 2 months) is usually due to seeding during the surgery. An acute presentation means emergent surgery is necessary. Even with surgery, it still has a 40% mortality.

Late type of PVE (> 2 months) has a subacute presentation. The infection often invades the annulus, and surgery is required. *S. epidermidis* is the culprit in 55–60% of the cases of PVE in the first year after surgery. If the infecting organism is viridans streptococci, antibiotics alone may cure the prosthetic valve infection. Better success is seen with porcine bioprosthesis, as opposed to metal valves.

Treatment of Bacterial Endocarditis

Treatment of native valve endocarditis:
- PCN-sensitive streptococcus (*S. bovis*): 2 weeks of PCN G or ampicillin + gentamicin or 4 weeks of either PCN/ampicillin, cefazolin, or ceftriaxone. Note: For this, vancomycin is less effective than beta-lactam antibiotics, so use only for severe PCN allergy. You can discharge reliable patients from the hospital on a once-daily IM dose of ceftriaxone.
- PCN-insensitive streptococcus (usually *Enterococcus faecalis*): the treatment is 4 weeks of gentamicin + either PCN G, ampicillin, or vancomycin, if PCN-allergic.
- Treat *S. aureus* endocarditis with oxacillin, vancomycin, or cefazolin. Again: If the *S. aureus* is methicillin-resistant, use vancomycin + gentamicin +/- rifampin.

Treatment of prosthetic valve endocarditis:
- Methicillin-resistant *Staph* (especially *Staph epidermidis*) requires vancomycin + rifampin + gentamicin—all 3—for 14 days, followed by vancomycin + rifampin for 4 weeks. The gentamicin prevents the emergence of resistance to rifampin. Remember: Both gentamicin and vancomycin are nephro- and ototoxic.
- *S. aureus*: Naf/ox or cefazolin + gentamicin for 5 days, followed by the beta-lactam for a total of 6 weeks.

COMMON ID SYNDROMES: CNS

Bacterial Meningitis

Overview

Acute Bacterial Meningitis—If suspected, do the following CSF tests: Gram-stain, C&S, cell count with differential, protein, and glucose.

Previously, CIE (counterimmunoelectrophoresis) or latex agglutination was used, but neither is cost-effective, therefore no longer indicated for initial workups. The culture results

notes

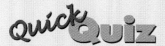
are the gold standard—unless the patient has been on prior antibiotics. CIE or latex agglutination tests the following: *H. influenzae*, pneumococcus, meningococcus, Group B *Strep*, *Klebsiella*, and *E. coli*. The sensitivity of these varies from 20% –90%.

Overall (see Table 2-5), *S. pneumoniae* is the most common cause of meningitis. Next is *Neisseria meningitidis*, then *Listeria monocytogenes*. Listerial meningitis becomes more prevalent again > 60 years old.

The main culprit in the meningococcal group is B (B for Bad, B for Bad). There are effective vaccines against A, C, Y, and W-135, but not type B (see pg 2-12 for meningococcemia).

In neonates (< 1 month old), think Gram-negative, group B *Strep* (*S. agalactiae*), and *Listeria*.

In children prior to 1990, *H. influenzae* was by far the most common cause. The HiB vaccine has had a wonderfully dramatic effect on this disease in the U.S. The incidence of *H. influenzae* infection has decreased from ~ 40% to ~ 2%!

Treatment of Bacterial Meningitis

In partially treated, Gram-positive meningitis, the bacteria stain poorly, and they may even look Gram-negative! A bloody tap (contaminated) has increased protein and decreased glucose.

Effective treatment requires an antibiotic that both crosses into the CSF and has bactericidal activity.

Antibiotics that cross into the CSF are:
- quinolones
- chloramphenicol
- TMP/SMX
- metronidazole

Those that cross into the CSF only with inflamed meninges are:
- PCN
- vancomycin
- 3rd gen cephalosporins
- aztreonam
- imipenem
- clindamycin

Clindamycin is effective in treating penicillin-resistant pneumococcal meningitis, and so probably does cross the blood-brain barrier with inflammation. Note that clindamycin is

used in the treatment of CNS toxoplasmosis, but this is a parenchymal disease and not a meningeal disease, so the drug does not have to cross the blood-brain barrier.

Those that do not cross well at any time are:
- erythromycin
- tetracycline
- aminoglycosides
- cefoxitin
- 1st gen cephalosporins

On the Boards, if you see any answers to meningitis questions with these last antibiotics in them, pick something else!

Start empiric treatment of meningitis while the spinal fluid Gram stain and/or culture results are pending. Note: If the lumbar puncture (LP) cannot be done immediately, start antibiotics anyway—even before the LP!

Meningitis in children and adults is empirically treated with ceftriaxone/cefotaxime (3rd gen cephalosporin) plus vancomycin (to cover resistant *S. pneumoniae*). Note: Resistant *S. pneumoniae* is more likely if the patient has recently been on antibiotics. Vancomycin is used because the *Strep* may be resistant to all penicillins and cephalosporins!

For empiric treatment of the elderly and neonates (< 3 months), add ampicillin (for *Listeria*), to the above treatment. So, these patients are often started on triple antibiotic therapy!

More specifically, in neonates (< 3 mo), use cefotaxime or ceftazidime as the 3rd gen cephalosporin because ceftriaxone may cause hyperbilirubinemia. (Remember: Ceftriaxone causes gallbladder sludge in adults.)

If you suspect any of the following, the empiric therapy may change:
- For presumed pneumococcal (especially if Gram stain is suspicious) meningitis, be sure to add vancomycin to the 3rd gen cephalosporin. Rifampin if vancomycin-allergic.
- Treat presumed meningococcal meningitis with high-dose PCN (3rd generation cephalosporin if PCN-allergic) and ensure contacts receive prophylaxis.
- The 3rd generation cephalosporins cover Gram-negative meningitis.

In AIDS, ALL, or Hodgkin disease, think *Cryptococcus* and do a cryptococcal antigen and/or India ink. Amebic meningitis should be the primary consideration when the meningitis patient has been swimming in brackish (cow ponds) water.

Aseptic Meningitis

Viruses are the most common cause of aseptic meningitis—these include enteroviruses and mosquito-borne arboviruses (West Nile virus!) in the summer/early fall, mumps in the spring (usually very rare today because of immunization although there was an outbreak in Iowa in 2006), and HSV-2. Suspect *Coccidioides* and *Histoplasma* in endemic areas (arid Southwest and Mississippi/Ohio River valleys, respectively). Cryptococcal meningitis is common in AIDS, Hodgkin disease, and ALL. Chronic neutrophilic meningitis is unusual—think of *Nocardia*, *Actinomyces*, or fungus as possible causes.

Manifestations of viral meningitis: headache, meningismus, and a nonfocal exam. CSF has lymphocytosis with usually < 250 cells/µL, and always < 2000 cells/µL, no organisms, normal to slightly elevated protein level, and normal glucose level (~ 60% of serum glucose).

When non-bacterial meningitis is suspected, do the same CSF tests as for acute meningitis and add: fungal serology, VDRL, acid-fast smear and culture, and either the India ink or cryptococcal antigen test.

CSF test results that make viral meningitis unlikely are CSF glucose < 40% of serum glucose, CSF protein > 150 g/dL, and CSF WBC: > 120 cells/ml.

Treat cryptococcal meningitis with IV amphotericin B + oral flucytosine (5-FC; 5-fluorocytosine), followed by oral fluconazole.

In AIDS patients, the CSF may have no WBCs in cryptococcal meningitis.

Eosinophilic Meningoencephalitis

Eosinophilic meningoencephalitis due to *Baylisascaris*, a nematode parasite of raccoons, has an increasing incidence because of increased raccoon populations in suburbia, particularly in California. Most infections occur in young children after they come in contact with raccoon feces in sandboxes. However, cases have also occurred in older adolescents and young adults. There is a profound eosinophilia in the CSF and multiple granuloma form in the brain tissue. There is no effective treatment at this time.

Other causes of eosinophilic meningitis include *Coccidioides* and *Angiostrongylus cantonensis*, the cause of eosinophilic meningitis in a honeymooner returning from Tahiti.

TB Meningitis

Tuberculous meningitis is sometimes manifested by cranial nerve palsies, especially the 6th cranial nerve. Look also for "basilar" enhancement on CT scan. Other causes of aseptic meningitis include spirochetal infection (secondary syphilis and Lyme disease).

Lyme Meningitis

Lyme meningitis can cause peripheral and cranial nerve palsies (especially of the 7th cranial nerve), so think of Lyme disease when a patient presents with Bell's palsy and/or foot drop and a suggestive history. Treat meningitis with ceftriaxone 2 gm qd x 21d. Treat Bell's palsy with oral agents alone. Alternative is high-dose PCN G.

Encephalitis

Acute encephalitis—the causes of most of the acute encephalitis cases are unknown! The most commonly identified causes of encephalitis in the U.S. are arboviruses (West Nile, La-Crosse, etc.).

HSV is responsible for the highest number of deaths due to encephalitis.

Spinal Epidural Abscess

Spinal epidural abscesses may be caused by either hematogenous spread or local extension (i.e., from osteomyelitis). *S. aureus* is the most common cause. Patients present with fever, spinal pain, and nerve compression problems. Do an MRI. CT is not as good as MRI because it is susceptible to bony artifacts. Drainage is required.

Neurosyphilis

Neurosyphilis—also see more about syphilis on pg 2-17. CSF-VDRL test is the test of choice; it is 100% specific, but only 50% sensitive. A positive test confirms neurosyphilis, but a negative test cannot be used to rule out neurosyphilis. CSF FTA-ABS is very sensitive; unfortunately, it is so sensitive that a positive result often reflects contamination of CSF with peripheral blood, so it is not used. Often, treatment has to be based on suspicion.

Table 2-5: Etiology of Meningitis in the United States						
0-2 month	%	3 mo to 15 years	%	Adult	%	Notes on > 60 years
Gram-neg (*E. coli* & *Klebsiella*)	20-30	***S. pneumoniae***	30-50	***S. pneumoniae***	30-50	*S. pneumoniae* *N. meningitidis*
Strep (Group B) (*S. agalactiae*)	40-50	***N. meningitidis***	10-35	***N. meningitidis***	10-35	See more: *Listeria* *E. coli* *H. influenzae* *Pseudomonas*
Listeria	2-10	***H. influenzae***	0-7	***Listeria***	2-11	
Staphylococci	2-5	Streptococci	2-4	Gram negative	1-10	
S. pneumoniae	0-5	Gram Negative	1-2	Streptococci	5	
H. influenzae	0-3	Staphylococci	1-2	Staphylococci	5	
N. meningitidis	0-1	*Listeria*	1-2	*H. influenzae*	1-3	

Remember, for the newborn and the adults > 60 yrs, empiric therapy now includes ceftriaxone, ampicillin (for *Listeria*), and vancomycin (for resistant *S. pneumoniae*).

notes

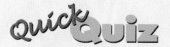

1) What are typical LP findings in a patient with viral meningitis?

2) A cranial nerve palsy should make you think of which 2 types of meningitis? (Hint: One is a spirochete and the other is a mycobacterium.) Which antibiotics do you give for empiric treatment of meningitis?

3) What virus type is the most common identified cause of acute encephalitis in the U.S.?

4) What virus is the most common cause of death due to encephalitis?

5) Multiple lesions on an MRI of the brain in an HIV-infected person should make you think of what organism?

6) What is the antibiotic of choice for diarrhea due to *E. coli* O157:H7? What about Travelers' diarrhea?

7) How do you diagnose *C. difficile* colitis?

Brain Abscess

Brain Abscess—Diagnosis: CT scan with contrast is the procedure of choice (> 95% sensitivity). If accessible, aspirate the abscess and give antibiotic treatment. Occasionally, you need to surgically excise the lesion. Lumbar puncture is absolutely contraindicated if signs of increased intracranial pressure are present—such as focal neurologic signs. Overall, the risk of herniation is as high as 20%

Cysticercosis (caused by ingesting the eggs of the pork tapeworm, *Taenia solium*) is the most common cause of brain lesions in developing countries, and imported cases are often seen in the U.S. Symptoms, especially seizures, occur when the cysticerci (larval forms of *T. solium*) die, causing an inflammatory reaction. *Toxoplasma* is the most likely etiologic agent if the patient is immunodeficient—especially if there are multiple lesions. It is usually due to a reactivation of dormant cysts.

Location of the abscess is often related to the source. Frontal lobe—think paranasal sinus: pneumococcus, *H. influenzae*, and anaerobes. Temporal or cerebellum—think middle ear: pneumococcus, *H. influenzae*, *S. aureus*, Gram-negative. Both frontal and parietal abscesses can be due to hematogenous spread from such things as lung infections and endocarditis.

Treatment of brain abscesses is always initially empiric:

• High-dose ampicillin or ceftriaxone + metronidazole to cover aerobes and anaerobes.

• PCN-allergic: give metronidazole + a 3rd generation cephalosporin.

• If you suspect *Enterobacteriaceae* (i.e., if ear focus), give a 3rd generation cephalosporin + metronidazole.

• If there was a neurosurgical procedure, penetrating head trauma, or acute endocarditis, think *S. aureus* and add vancomycin (high incidence of MRSA).

Nocardia pulmonary disease can spread and cause focal lesions in the brain. It is also a rare cause of neutrophilic aseptic meningitis (see just above).

COMMON ID SYNDROMES: GASTROINTESTINAL

E. coli is the most common cause of bacterial diarrhea (usually without blood or WBCs) affecting both the resident children and travelers in developing countries. There is an enterohemorrhagic *E. coli* (serotype O157:H7), which causes localized outbreaks of hemorrhagic colitis, TTP, and HUS (hemolytic uremic syndrome)—usually after eating undercooked beef or unpasteurized milk. Do not treat diarrhea caused by *E. coli* O157:H7 with antibiotics because you increase the risk of HUS.

Vibrios—think seafood and shellfish. *V. cholerae* 01 (causes cholera) is occasionally associated with gulf coast crabs. The *non*-01 *V. cholera*, *V. parahaemolyticus*, and other *Vibrios* are even more frequent causes of shellfish-associated diarrhea. These are usually self-limited. *Vibrio vulnificus* causes skin infections and sepsis, especially in the setting of immunocompromise or chronic liver disease (see pg 2-47).

Fecal WBCs suggest an invasive-type bacterial etiology and are evident in *Shigella*, *Salmonella*, *Campylobacter jejuni*, *Yersinia enterocolitica*, and amebic GI infections. But remember: They are also seen in IBD. All of these organisms can be found on C&S, and *Vibrios* additionally can be found on stool C&S and O&P. So, do a fecal WBC and stool C&S and O&P if you need to work up a diarrhea. See Gastroenterology section for more on diarrhea.

Antibiotic-associated colitis is caused by *Clostridium difficile* (antibiotic-associated diarrhea is usually just a side effect of the medicine). Symptoms can occur up to 3 weeks after the antibiotics are stopped. To diagnose, do a stool assay for the *Clostridium difficile* cytotoxin. A toxin assay is required because 5% of healthy persons have *C. difficile* in their stool and not all of the *C. difficile* organisms produce the cytotoxin. Treatment: Stop the antibiotics and give 7–10 days of metronidazole or oral vancomycin. Other treatments are bacitracin, rifampin, or bile-binding resins (e.g., cholestyramine), which bind the toxin. Usual treatment is metronidazole, because it is generally just as effective as oral vancomycin yet much less expensive. Recent data suggest that oral vancomycin is superior to metronidazole for severe disease. Relapse rate on either drug is ~ 30%. This is usually due to the spores becoming active; just repeat the same treatment! Use bacitracin, rifampin, and cholestyramine as adjuncts in complicated cases. Rifaximin and nitazoxanide have been used for refractory disease although they are not FDA approved as yet for this indication.

Cryptosporidia is known to cause prolonged diarrhea in AIDS patients and a self-limited diarrhea in travelers. It is found with acid-fast stains of the stool (small, round, red organisms on a green background). Animals (including humans) are the reservoirs.

Enterotoxigenic *E. coli* is the usual cause of Travelers' diarrhea. Prophylaxis with bismuth subsalicylate (Pepto-Bismol®, Kaopectate®) qid or with daily quinolone. Treatment: Mild: Loperamide + single-dose quinolone. Severe: Same except add quinolone bid x 3 days.

Note: Start cultures for *Shigella* (usually *Shigella sonnei*!) as soon as possible after the bowel movement because *Shigella* dies soon after exposure to air.

Viral causes of diarrhea—rotavirus is frequently found in children. It is the most important cause of severe diarrhea in infants and easily evident in their stools. Noroviruses (formerly known as Norwalk-type viruses) are associated with clams and oysters, causing "winter vomiting disease," but it can also be water-borne. Identify noroviruses with the ELISA test. Look for outbreaks on cruise ships!

Treatment—If there are fecal WBCs, do a stool C&S and O&P, but fluoroquinolones or TMP/SMX are usually given empirically, although antibiotics may prolong *Salmonella* infection. Do not give antimotility agents for any diarrhea when there are fecal WBCs. *Campylobacter* is resistant to TMP/SMX, so give erythromycin or quinolones instead. Prolonged, intermittent diarrhea with malaise and flatus suggests giardiasis or *Cyclospora*.

COMMON ID SYNDROMES: GENITOURINARY INFECTIONS & STD

Note

There are many causes of STD. Know the treatment of all STDs! Many STDs have similar manifestations, consisting of genital ulcerations with regional adenopathy (gonorrhea does not have these).

GU Infections with Genital Ulcerations

Workup of genital ulcer (or ulcers) with regional lymphadenopathy: Serologic tests for syphilis, culture or antigen test for HSV, culture for *H. ducreyi* (on chocolate agar), and, if indicated by history and physical exam, you may need to do LGV titers or biopsy the nodes to look for granulomas (Donovan bodies).

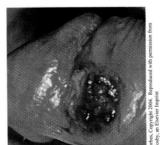

Image 2-35: Syphilis - typical primary chancre in coronal sulcus

Forbes, Copyright 2004. Reproduced with permission from Mosby, an Elsevier Imprint

With syphilis, the ulcer is usually single, clean with raised borders, and painless (See Image 2-35). Patients with syphilis also typically have large painless lymph nodes (see pg 2-17 for more on syphilis).

HSV presents with tender grouped vesicles. It may or may not have regional adenopathy.

Treat with oral acyclovir for the initial episode. You may also try this for severe, recurrent disease.

Haemophilus ducreyi causes chancroid in which there are tender genital papules, which become painful purulent ulcers with irregular borders. There is associated, very painful lymphadenopathy, which rapidly becomes fluctuant and ruptures. Treat with one dose of ceftriaxone (250 mg IM) or oral azithromycin 1.0 gm oral single dose, or ciprofloxacin 500 mg bid x 3 d or erythromycin 500 mg tid x 7d.

Chlamydia trachomatis causes lymphogranuloma venereum (LGV). It starts with a painless papule, which goes on to ulcerate and then disappears in 1–3 weeks. Inguinal adenopathy develops 2–6 weeks later. In LGV, the adenopathy may bulge over either side of the inguinal ligament, and fistulae sometime develop. Usual treatment is doxycycline 100 mg bid x 21 d. Erythromycin 500 mg tid x 21 d is effective as well.

Granuloma inguinale ("Donovanosis") is rare. *Klebsiella granulomatis* (formerly *Calymmatobacterium granulomatis*) is the causative Gram-negative organism that produces terrible looking genital ulcers, which are painless! Treat with doxycycline 100 mg bid x 21 d or until well healed—may take 1 month. TMP/SMX also used. Erythromycin if pregnant.

PID

PID can be caused by *N. gonorrhoeae*, *Chlamydia*, and normal vaginal flora (usually anaerobes). Oral contraceptives reduce the risk of severely symptomatic PID caused by gonococci, but "silent" PID has the same incidence of sequelae (infertility) as does that associated with peritoneal signs! Cervical cultures are not reliable for PID. Occasionally, PID patients get a perihepatitis (Fitz-Hugh-Curtis syndrome) with mild LFT abnormalities; this has been caused by both *N. gonorrhea* and *Chlamydia*. Because of the rate of fluoroquinolone-resistant gonorrhea, fluoroquinolones are no longer recommended.

Outpatient Treatment for PID:
• Ceftriaxone 250 mg IM, then doxycycline 100 mg bid x 14 d +/- metronidazole 500 mg bid x 14 d OR
• Cefoxitin 2 g IM and probenecid 1 g x 1 plus doxycycline +/- metronidazole OR
• Other parenteral cephalosporin (ceftizoxime or cefotaxime) plus doxycycline +/- metronidazole

Inpatient Treatment for PID (Either of 2 recommended parenteral regimens):
• Cefotetan 2 grams IV q 12 hours (or cefoxitin 2 gm IV q 6 hours) and doxycycline 100 mg orally or IV q 12 hours OR
• Clindamycin 900 mg IV q 8 hours + gentamicin.

notes

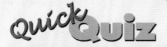

Quick Quiz

1) What is the most important cause of severe diarrhea in infants?
2) What type of viral diarrhea is associated with clams? How would you diagnose it?
3) *Chlamydia* cervicitis typically has what type of discharge?
4) What do Gram-negative intracellular diplococci imply in a smear of a discharge from urethritis?
5) Fever, arthralgia, and oligoarthritis in a young sexually active woman should make you think of what organism?
6) Initially, do you treat or just test the asymptomatic sexual partner of a person with gonococcal urethritis? With non-GC urethritis?
7) What kind of skin lesions do patients with gonococcemia get?

• An alternative to these 2 is ampicillin/sulbactam and doxycycline.

Again: When treating gonorrhea, always cover for *Chlamydia*. Tubo-ovarian abscesses require inpatient, intravenous antibiotic therapy—same as the inpatient PID choices above, and note that ampicillin/sulbactam + doxycycline is also recommended for tubo-ovarian abscesses.

Follow up with patients treated for chlamydial infections with a test for cure at 3 weeks.

Cervicitis

Cervicitis is usually caused by *Chlamydia* (especially if the discharge is mucopurulent), but also *N. gonorrhoeae*, herpes, and papillomaviruses. Because *Chlamydia* is intracellular, you must have cervical cells for a valid smear/culture (so scrape or use a brush). *Chlamydia* cervicitis commonly has a mucopurulent discharge. Gram stain of cervical discharge is only 50% sensitive for the gonococcus, so a negative smear does not exclude gonococci.

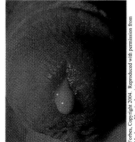

Image 2-36: Gonorrhea

Forbes, Copyright 2004. Reproduced with permission from Mosby, an Elsevier Imprint.

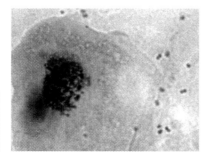

Image 2-37: Gram-negative diplococci – these are extracellular. Require intracellular for Dx.

Urethritis

Urethritis—gonococcal or nongonococcal. With GC urethritis, the patient virtually always has a purulent discharge, but make the diagnosis from either positive culture results or the finding of Gram-negative intracellular (within PMNs) diplococci on Gram stain (See Image 2-36 and Image 2-37).

Otherwise, consider it non-GC urethritis, which is usually due to *Chlamydia trachomatis* and, less frequently, *Ureaplasma urealyticum*, *Trichomonas vaginalis*, or HSV. For 35% of cases, the cause is unknown.

In the non-GC urethritis, the patients usually have a clear urethral discharge, and a Gram stain shows WBCs and no bacteria. Gonococcal urethritis has a shorter incubation period (2–6 days vs. 1–4 weeks for *Chlamydia*) and produces a more purulent and more productive discharge.

In all of these patients, check a VDRL and, if negative, repeat it in 2 months (in case the syphilis was incubating when blood for the first test was drawn). Offer HIV testing to all urethritis patients.

Treatment of urethritis:

1) Treat non-GC urethritis with azithromycin 1 gm orally in a single dose or doxycycline 100 mg bid x 7 d. Use erythromycin for pregnant women. Azithromycin 1 gm orally x 1 dose appears as effective as doxycycline, but it is much more expensive. Levofloxacin and ofloxacin are also effective.

2) GC urethritis. There is about a 20% incidence of gonococcal resistance to penicillin and about the same to tetracycline. Also, because there is often a coinfection with *Chlamydia*, always cover *U. urealyticum* and *Chlamydia* with treatment of gonococcal urethritis. The standard treatment protocol for GC urethritis: For uncomplicated gonococcal urethritis or mucopurulent cervicitis, give 1 dose of cefixime 400 mg orally or ceftriaxone (Rocephin®) 125 mg IM, followed by 7 days of doxycycline 100 mg bid or azithromycin 1 gm x single dose. Spectinomycin 2 gm IM may be substituted for ceftriaxone in penicillin-allergic patients, but know that spectinomycin does not cure pharyngeal gonococcal disease (and also it is not currently available in the U.S., but the guidelines list it as the alternative in cephalosporin allergic patients!). Quinolone resistance is too high in the U.S., and thus they are no longer recommended for treatment of gonorrhea.

Always treat the sexual partners of patients with either type of urethritis, even if they are not symptomatic! And always treat suspected cases immediately—don't wait for C&S results!

Disseminated Gonococcemia

Disseminated gonococcemia: [Know!] Patients present with a fever, arthralgias, and occasionally oligoarthritis—usually of the knee or ankle. Tenosynovitis is common and frequently asked about. The patient typically has muscle aches and a

notes

rash with a few lesions that are papular with hemorrhage into the papules (i.e., very red papules). Notes: Gonococcus-associated arthritis is asymmetric; gonococcemia is more likely and more severe during menstruation; pili on the organism are associated with increased virulence.

Gram stain and culture have a very low yield (10%) from the lesions, but if you swab all orifices, there is an 85% yield. Even though the lesions have a low yield, they should still be tested, because similar lesions can be caused by other disseminated diseases, such as *Staph* endocarditis (which does have a positive Gram stain and C+S).

Treat patients diagnosed with gonococcemia (including tenosynovitis) with a 3rd generation cephalosporin (ceftriaxone, ceftizoxime, or cefotaxime). Pending culture and sensitivity, single-dose azithromycin, ofloxacin/levofloxacin, or doxycycline are included to cover for *Chlamydia*.

Epididymitis

Epididymitis is an inflammation of the epididymis—a convoluted duct on the posterior of the testicle. It is usually caused by infection [Know]:

• *Enterobacteriaceae*, especially *E. coli*, in prepubertal boys and men > 35 years old.
• STD pathogens in sexually active men < 35 years—especially *C. trachomatis*.

Vaginitis

1) Bacterial vaginosis is a clinical syndrome resulting from the replacement of the normal H_2O_2-producing *lactobacillus* in the vagina with high concentrations of anaerobic bacteria (*Mobiluncus*), *Gardnerella vaginalis*, and *Mycoplasma hominis*. There is a thin, "skim milk," scanty, bad-smelling, non-irritating discharge that has 2 identifying features: clue cells (an epithelial cell with many adherent bacteria) and a fishy odor when mixed with KOH (+whiff/sniff test). There is no *cervical* discharge.

• Treatment is usually metronidazole—oral (500 mg bid x 7 d) or vaginal gel (.75% bid x 5 d).
• Alternative therapy is clindamycin oral (300 mg bid x 7 d) or vaginal cream (2% bid x 7 d).

Treatment guidelines have changed for pregnant women!
• Metronidazole 500 mg bid x 7 days or
• Metronidazole 250 mg tid x 7 d or
• Clindamycin 300 mg orally bid x 7 d.
• Creams are not recommended in pregnancy.

The reason to treat systemically is that there is a much higher risk of preterm labor and delivery than complication from a short course of therapy with metronidazole or clindamycin. The male sex partner does not need to be treated.

2) Vulvovaginal candidiasis (VVC) is usually caused by *Candida albicans*. It presents with adherent white plaques with an erythematous base. Treatment:

• Uncomplicated VVC in a non-pregnant patient: clotrimazole or miconazole OTC vaginal creams or clotrimazole 500 mg tablet intravaginally are the least expensive effective treatments. Oral azoles are equally effective—especially oral fluconazole 150 mg one-time dose!
• Treat pregnant patients only with the azole creams for 7 days.
• A subgroup of patients have recurrent VVC, which just does not go away, and does not have an optimum treatment. Weekly topical clotrimazole or oral fluconazole 150 mg one-time dose is effective. Conduct HIV testing in women with recurrent or persistent VVC.

3) *Trichomonas vaginalis* infection causes a vaginitis in women, but men are usually asymptomatic. 1 week to 1 month incubation period. Trich vaginitis often presents with a profuse, thin, frothy, yellow-green, bad-smelling discharge (which, like bacterial vaginosis, has a + whiff test!), vaginal erythema, and a strawberry cervix. Be able to identify the flagellated organism on wet mount—which is only 50% sensitive. DIF antibody staining is 70–90% sensitive. The vaginal pH is < 4.5 in the normal secretions and in yeast vaginitis. It is > 5.0 in trichomoniasis and bacterial vaginosis.

Treat trich vaginitis with metronidazole 2.0 grams single dose or tinidazole 2 grams single dose. Even though this is the best treatment, it is only moderately effective. If pregnant, recommendations say it is OK to give one-time dose of 2 gram metronidazole.

Urinary Tract Infection

Acute urethral syndrome (dysuria, frequency, and pyuria) is most commonly caused by *E. coli* and *Chlamydia trachomatis*. *S. saprophyticus* causes cystitis in young women—this is a coagulase-negative staphylococcus.

The symptoms of acute urethral syndrome may be due to either urethritis, vaginitis, or cystitis. In women, sexual intercourse can cause *E. coli* to be pushed up the urethra, predisposing them for an acute cystitis. Besides sexual activity, other UTI-predisposing factors in women include spermicide-diaphragm use and an inherited abnormality called Lewis non-secretor phenotype.

UTIs are rare in men and are not associated with male sexual activity, except in homosexuals. In non-homosexual men, UTIs are usually a result of an abnormality in the urinary tract such as obstruction and ureterovesical reflux from prostatic hypertrophy. Both men and women with DM, neurogenic bladders, or indwelling catheters have an increased frequency of UTIs.

Diagnosis criteria have changed. Urine cultures are no longer required on all young women with symptoms of an acute UTI. If there are no complicating factors, pyuria alone is an indication to treat.

Treatment of UTIs:
• routine UTI: TMP/SMX for 3 days. (TMP/SMX is more effective than amoxicillin).
• uncomplicated pyelonephritis: the treatment is oral TMP/SMX for 14 days.

notes

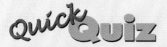

Quick Quiz

1) What are the most common causes of epididymitis by age group?

2) What is the treatment for pregnant women with bacterial vaginosis?

3) What serologic test would you order for recurrent VVC?

4) In a healthy young woman, what is the length of therapy for a routine UTI?

5) Asymptomatic bacteriuria is always treated with antibiotics in which group of patients? Why?

6) What type of bacteria are commonly found in shellfish? Who are especially susceptible?

7) A fish tank cleaner comes in with nonhealing skin ulcerations in a lymphatic distribution. What is the prime suspect? How is it treated?

8) Acute osteomyelitis is usually caused by what organism? What organism do you suspect in an IVDA? In SS patients?

9) A patient you suspect has osteomyelitis has a negative bone scan. Do you now do an open bone Bx?

10) What is the most common means of spreading infections in the ICU?

• complicated pyelonephritis (includes pregnant patients! For Tx, see below): IV ampicillin + gentamicin, TMP/SMX, fluoroquinolones, or 3rd generation cephalosporins. Use gentamicin alone if the Gram stain shows no Gram-positive cocci but, because of toxicity issues, gentamicin is being used less commonly and has largely been supplanted by quinolone or 3rd generation therapy. Follow up with urine analysis after antibiotic treatment. Fluoroquinolones are alternate therapy for complicated or recurrent cystitis or pyelonephritis.

Organisms to know: *Proteus* infections are associated with stones (i.e., do a KUB to check for stones). Group B *Strep* (*S. agalactiae*) infections are seen in pregnancy.

Pregnant women (Know!): Treat asymptomatic bacteriuria in pregnant women (1/3 go on to pyelonephritis!), neutropenic patients, diabetics, and transplant patients. Also, always admit and treat pregnant patients with pyelonephritis as a complicated pyelonephritis (above). Pregnancy-safe antibiotics to use for UTI/pyelonephritis are ampicillin, cephalosporins, and TMP/SMX, but do not give TMP/SMX in late pregnancy or to early nursing mothers because it might cause kernicterus in the child. Do not use tetracy-cline/doxycycline or quinolones.

There is an increased frequency of urinary tract infections in patients with DM, sickle cell disease, hyperparathyroidism, or gout. In the last two, the UTI is secondary to stone formation and obstruction. UTIs are the most common nosocomial infections. With normal catheter care, most indwelling urinary catheters stay sterile up to 7 days. They used to be changed out after 7 days of use, but now are changed only when the patient has signs or symptoms of infection.

Pyelonephritis in older men is often caused by bladder outlet obstruction due to prostatic hypertrophy. Be especially on the lookout for *Enterococcus*, as well as the usual Gram-negative organisms!

COMMON ID SYNDROMES: SOFT TISSUE, BONE, & JOINT INFECTIONS

Vibrio are found especially in shellfish. *V. vulnificus* causes large hemorrhagic bullae, followed by necrosis and lymphadenopathy +/- septicemia. Patients who are immunocompromised or have chronic liver disease are especially susceptible.

Mycobacterium marinum is also called "fish tank bacillus." It causes non-healing skin ulceration in people who work around fish tanks. Infection may present as a single granuloma, but the organism often invades the lymphatics and can cause a series of lesions over a lymph vessel similar to the lesions seen in sporotrichosis. Lesions tend to localize in the distal extremities because the organism does not grow well at body temperature. DDx: Look for acid-fast bacilli in the lesion biopsy. Treat with ethambutol + rifampin or clarithromycin + rifampin.

Erysipelothrix rhusiopathiae is another cause of skin infection in fishermen and meat handlers. Treat with PCN G, ampicillin, or fluoroquinolones.

Impetigo presents as honey-colored crusts over lesions. *Strep pyogenes* is a common cause, often in combination with *S. aureus*. Remember: *S. pyogenes* also causes scarlet fever, a type of toxic shock syndrome (TSS), pharyngitis, and rheumatic heart disease.

Osteomyelitis—acute vs. chronic. Both have infection, but only chronic osteomyelitis has necrotic bone. Acute is usually caused by *S. aureus*. Think *Pseudomonas* in an IV drug abuser, especially if the infection involves the vertebrae or pelvis. Think *Salmonella* in Sickle Cell (SS) patients. Streptococci are virtually never a cause of osteomyelitis! Blood cultures are usually (2/3!) positive in acute osteomyelitis. A negative pyrophosphate bone scan excludes osteomyelitis, but positive scans may also be seen with other infections and with fractures. Usually, you see x-ray changes only with chronic osteomyelitis.

With sinus tract osteomyelitis, C&S of the sinus tract drainage is sufficient if you find *S. aureus*, but it is not sufficient otherwise—must use bone biopsy/scraping.

With suspected spinal osteomyelitis, do a needle biopsy as the first diagnostic procedure.

Except for small bone disease, you must remove the necrotic bone before a chronic osteomyelitis can be cured with antibiotics.

Prosthetic joints—1% get infected. Presentation is usually chronic. X-rays usually show bony changes, but a bone scan may be needed. You must perform a joint aspiration to de-

notes

termine the infecting organism. Coagulase-negative staphylococci (e.g., *S. epidermidis*) are the most common organisms recovered.

COMMON ID SYNDROMES: NOSOCOMIAL INFECTIONS

Order of frequency: UTI > post-op wound infection > pneumonia.

Nosocomial pneumonia is usually bacterial and has the highest mortality rate of all the nosocomial infections (1/3 if bacteremic; 1/2 if Gram-negative bacteremic!) It is usually caused by Gram-negative organisms; next most frequently, *Staph aureus*. Resistance may develop quickly if only a single broad-spectrum antibiotic is used. If there is an outbreak of bacterial pneumonia (or almost any illness) in the ICU, the most likely vector of transmission is the hands of the ICU workers.

Catheter-related infections—there are 3 types, and all 3 can cause bacteremia/fungemia: 1) asymptomatic, 2) localized, and 3) septic thrombophlebitis (rarest—see *Candida* on pg 2-19). Secondary endocarditis is more likely to occur in patients with catheters that extend into the heart. IV lines become infected after ~ 3 days! Metal needles are less likely than plastic angiocatheters to become infected. IV catheter infections are usually due to *S. epidermidis* and *S. aureus*. Some other causes are *Candida*, *Corynebacterium jeikeium* (especially in bone marrow transplant units) and Gram-negative rods.

Treatment: Remove catheter and give antibiotic therapy for 2 weeks. Septic thrombophlebitis often requires removal of the affected vein. If there is Gram-positive septicemia, start with vancomycin in case it is methicillin-resistant. Exception—if there is a Gram-positive bacteremia in a patient with a Hickman or Broviac, you can try to treat with antibiotics for 2–4 weeks without removing the catheter. Again, start with vancomycin until culture results are back.

notes

The following material is to assist you in integrating the information you have just reviewed in this section. These are purposely NOT Board-style questions since they are meant to cover a lot of material in minimal space. MedStudy does have Board-style Q&A products separately available in book and software formats.

SINGLE BEST ANSWER

This is a set of questions in which there is more than one answer for many of the questions, but you must pick the single best answer.

1)   A. Infections caused by *Nocardia* and *Listeria*, fungi, and protozoa.
     B. Infections from encapsulated organisms (*H. flu*, pneumococcus, meningococcus).
     C. Asthma and recurrent pneumonia.
     D. Infections caused by Gram-negative organisms, *S. aureus*, and fungi.
     E. None of the above.

Which of the following cause an increased tendency for the above infections?

1. Splenectomy.
2. Neutropenia/granulocytopenia.
3. C1 deficiency.
4. C8 deficiency.
5. Multiple myeloma.
6. IgA deficiency.
7. T-cell deficiency

[1 (B. This is effectively a humoral deficiency. Babesiosis and malaria are also much worse in splenectomized patients.) 2 (D) 3 (B) 4 (B. Same infections are seen in humoral deficiency. Patients with late complement deficiency are especially susceptible to meningococcal infections.) 5 (B. MM causes a humoral deficiency.) 6 (C. IgA deficiency also is suggested with recurrent giardiasis.) 7 (A)]

---

2) Post-transplant infections
     A. Within first month post-transplant.
     B. Within 6 weeks post-transplant.
     C. 1–4 months post-transplant.
     D. 2–6 months post-transplant.
     E. After 4 months post-transplant.

1. *Cryptococcus neoformans*.
2. Nosocomial infections.
3. T-cell deficiency associated infections.
4. Viruses.
5. HSV reactivation.

[1 (E) 2 (A) 3 (C; especially CMV) 4 (D. The viruses are also due to T-cell deficiency, but all except CMV tend to occur a little later than the other T-cell deficiency infections.) 5 (B. This overlaps with the nosocomial infections but is easy to differentiate.)]

---

3) Infections caused by Gram-positive organisms:
     A. *Staph aureus*.
     B. *Staph epidermidis*.
     C. *Strep pyogenes*.
     D. *Strep pneumoniae*.
     E. *Strep agalactiae*.
     F. *Enterococcus faecalis*.
     G. *Listeria monocytogenes*.
     H. *Corynebacterium diphtheriae*.
     I. *Corynebacterium jeikeium* (JK).
     J. *Bacillus anthracis*.
     K. *Bacillus cereus*.
     L. *Clostridium septicum*.

1. Painless black eschars.
2. Sepsis after a TURP.
3. Severe resistant infection seen in bone marrow transplant units.
4. Associated with GI malignancy.
5. Most common cause of bacteremia after prosthetic valve surgery.
6. Most common cause of bacteremia in IV drug abusers and dialysis patients.
7. Most common cause of IV catheter-related bacteremia.
8. Pharyngitis with high-grade fever, tender cervical lymphadenopathy, and exudative tonsils.
9. M protein.
10. Alpha toxin.
11. TSS with negative blood cultures.
12. Hoarseness, sore throat, and low-grade fever.

[1 (J) 2 (F) 3 (I) 4 (L) 5 (B) 6 (A) 7 (B) 8 (C) 9 (C. The major protein on the *S. pyogenes* cell surface is the "M protein." The M protein defines which strains are rheumatogenic, cause glomerulonephritis, toxigenic for toxic shock syndrome, etc.) 10 (L; and all other *Clostridia*) 11(A) 12 (H)]

---

4) Infections caused by acid-fast bacteria:
     A. *M. avium-intracellulare*.
     B. *M. marinum*.
     C. *M. tuberculosis*.
     D. *Nocardia asteroides*.
     E. *Cryptosporidium*.
     F. *Isospora belli*.

1. Pleural effusion has a high lymphocyte count, no bacteria, and a low glucose.
2. Associated with thin-walled cavitary lung lesions and brain lesions.
3. Causes strings of nonhealing ulcers over lymph channels.
4. Common cause of chronic diarrhea in AIDS patients. Small and round.
5. Lymphadenitis in children.
6. Common cause of chronic diarrhea in AIDS patients. Large and oval.

[1 (C) 2 (D) 3 (B. This is called the "fish-tank bacillus.") 4 (E) 5 (A; as does *M. scrofulaceum*) 6 (F)]

---

5) Match the facts with the following diseases:
   A. Brucellosis.
   B. Tularemia.
   C. Plague.
   D. Bartonellosis.
   E. Legionellosis.
   F. Typhoid fever.
   G. Rocky mountain spotted fever.
   H. Leptospirosis.

1. Presenting symptoms: pneumonia, confusion, and diarrhea.
2. Carriers of this disease often have seeding in the gallstones.
3. Maculopapular-to-petechial rash. Fever and arthralgias.
4. Causes abortions in affected cattle; does not cause abortions in humans.
5. Hunter gets constitutional symptoms, localized suppurative lymphadenopathy, and no skin signs.
6. Hunter gets constitutional symptoms, localized lymphadenopathy, and localized ulceration and diffuse rash.
7. Suspect this in a hepatitis with the bilirubin disproportionately high compared to the liver enzymes.
8. Rapid onset of febrile hemolytic anemia.

[1 (E) 2 (F) 3 (G) 4 (A) 5 (C) 6 (B) 7 (H) 8 (D)]

6) Syphilis
   A. Primary infection.
   B. Secondary infection.
   C. Tertiary infection.
   D. None of the above.

1. Variable mucocutaneous lesions.
2. Diffuse involvement.
3. CNS lues.
4. Painless chancre.
5. Lesions on the palms and soles.
6. General lymphadenopathy.
7. Aortitis.
8. Argyll Robertson pupil.

[1 (B) 2 (B. Secondary infection is characterized by diffuse rash, lymphadenopathy, meningovascular disease, etc.) 3 (C) 4 (A) 5 (B) 6 (B. The multiple and various skin lesions and generalized lymphadenopathy occur in secondary syphilis.) 7 (C) 8 (C. CNS disease and aortitis occur in tertiary syphilis.)]

7) Fungi:
   A. Yeasts.
   B. Molds.
   C. Dimorphic fungi.

1. Spores.
2. *Candida.*
3. *Histoplasma.*
4. Dermatophytes.
5. *Cryptococcus.*
6. *Coccidioides.*

7. Most likely to cause systemic disease in the immunocompetent host.
8. *Blastomyces.*
9. *Sporothrix.*

[1 (B) 2 (A) 3 (C) 4 (B) 5 (A) 6 (C) 7 (C) 8 (C) 9 (C)]

8) Fungi:
   A. Dermatophytosis.
   B. Chronic mucocutaneous candidiasis.
   C. Sporotrichosis.
   D. Histoplasmosis.
   E. Blastomycosis.
   F. Cryptococcal disease. Coccidioidomycosis.
   H. Candidiasis.
   I. Mucormycosis.

1. Pulmonary infiltrates, constitutional symptoms, crusted skin lesions.
2. Interstitial pneumonia, palate ulcers, and splenomegaly.
3. Cotton wool patches on the retina.
4. Associated with a T-cell abnormality.
5. Suspect as a cause of meningitis in an AIDS patient.
6. Skin nodules along the lymphatic channels.
7. Mississippi and Ohio River valleys.
8. Associated with polyglandular deficiency.
9. Black lesion on the nose of a diabetic.
10. Flu symptoms in Arizona.

[1 (E) 2 (D) 3 (H) 4 (B) 5 (F) 6 (C. Remember that patients with this disease often work around soil—e.g., gardeners.) 7 (D) 8 (B) 9 (I) 10 (G)]

9) Treatments for parasites:
   A. Chloroquine.
   B. Spiramycin.
   C. Mefloquine.
   D. Chloroquine followed by primaquine.
   E. Pyrimethamine and trisulfapyrimidine.
   F. Exchange transfusion followed by clindamycin + quinine.
   G. TMP/SMX.

1. Ocular toxoplasmosis.
2. Duffy RBC antigen.
3. AIDS patient presents with a dry cough and shortness of breath. Chest x-ray shows diffuse infiltrates.
4. *P. ovale.*
5. AIDS patient with diarrhea. Acid-fast stain positive with large oval organisms.
6. *P. malariae.*
7. Banana gametocyte on peripheral blood smear.
8. Several *Plasmodium* parasites in one cell.
9. Febrile hemolytic anemia in an asplenic patient who is confused and combative. On peripheral smear are intracellular parasites with the form of a tetrad.

[1 (E; or pyrimethamine and sulfadiazine) 2 (D. The Duffy RBC antigen is the site of attachment for *P. vivax*.) 3 (G) 4 (D. Both *P. vivax* and *P. ovale* form hypnozoites in the liver. Primaquine destroys these forms.) 5 (G) 6 (A) 7 (C) 8 (C. *P. falciparum* can be treated with chloroquine only if it is chloroquine-sensitive. If not, it can be treated with PO quinine sulfate and either pyrimethamine + sulfadoxine (Fansidar®), doxycycline, or clindamycin. If the patient is unable to tolerate PO drugs, IV quinine gluconate and IV clindamycin are used.)
9 (F. This is babesiosis. Treat moderate infections with clindamycin + quinine or atovaquone + azithromycin.)]

10) A. *Giardia lamblia*
    B. *Trichomonas vaginalis.*
    C. *Trypanosoma.*
    D. *Leishmania.*
    E. All of the above.
    F. None of the above.

1. Megacolon.
2. Kala-azar.
3. Protozoa.
4. Duodenal infection.
5. Achalasia.
6. Sleeping sickness.
7. String test.
8. Flagellates.

[1 (C) 2 (D. Kala-azar is also known as visceral leishmaniasis. It is caused by *L. donovani*.) 3 (E) 4 (A) 5 (C. Achalasia, megaesophagus, and megacolon can be results of *T. cruzi* infection.) 6 (C. *T. brucei* is transmitted via the tsetse fly.) 7 (A) 8 (E. The flagellates, which include all of the above organisms, are a type of protozoa. However, note that even though *Leishmania* are included in the protozoan class of flagellates, they are not flagellated in their infectious forms.)]

11) Helminths: Trematodes (flukes)
    A. *Clonorchis sinensis.*
    B. *Schistosoma haematobium.*
    C. *Schistosoma mansoni.*
    D. *Schistosoma japonicum.*
    E. All of the above.
    F. None of the above.

1. Infects the bladder.
2. Caused by eating raw fish; causes biliary obstruction.
3. Found in Asia.
4. Found in South America.
5. Endemic in Japan and Korea.

[1 (B) 2 (A) 3 (A, D) 4 (C; also in Africa and the Middle East) 5 (A)]

12) Helminths: Nematodes
    A. *Ascaris lumbricoides.*
    B. *Enterobius.*
    C. *Necator americanus.*
    D. *Trichuris.*
    E. *Trichinella spiralis.*
    F. *Wuchereria bancrofti.*
    G. *Strongyloides.*

1. Rectal itching.
2. Replicates in the body.
3. Elephantiasis.
4. Frequency of infection in the U. S. is 4%.
5. Pinworm.
6. Infection often lasts for decades.
7. Hookworm. Causes weakness and fatigue.
8. Whipworm.
9. Organism is usually found in pork.

[1 (B) 2 (G. *Strongyloides* is virtually the only helminth which replicates in the body.) 3 (F) 4 (E; per autopsy findings.) 5 (B) 6 (G) 7 (C) 8 (D) 9 (E)]

13) Herpes viruses:
    A. Herpes zoster.
    B. Herpes simplex.
    C. Cytomegalovirus (CMV).
    D. Epstein-Barr virus.

1. C-section is recommended if mother has active lesions at the time of delivery.
2. Chorioretinitis in an AIDS patient.
3. Most common cause of blindness in industrialized nations.
4. Post-transplant patient presents with hepatitis, colitis, encephalitis, and adrenalitis.
5. Heterophil antibody titers positive.
6. Patient presents with altered mental status and left arm paralysis.
7. Atypical lymphocytes.
8. Inclusion bodies.

[1 (B. Remember that this is single best answer. The other viruses do not cause an infection that requires a C-section, while a vaginal herpes infection at the time of delivery does.) 2 (C) 3 (B) 4 (C) 5 (D) 6 (B) 7 (D) 8 (C. Also remember: Herpes virus skin infections are diagnosed by finding multinucleated giant cells on the Tzanck test.)]

14) A. Rhinovirus.
    B. Respiratory syncytial virus.
    C. Parvovirus.
    D. Rubeola.
    E. Rubella.
    F. Hepatitis C.

1. High chance of congenital defect if acquired during the first trimester of pregnancy.
2. Koplik's spots.
3. Diagnosed by an ELISA test on nasal secretions.
4. "Slapped-cheek" appearance.
5. Treat with ribavirin and interferon alpha.
6. Measles.
7. German measles.
8. A common cause of URIs.
9. Giant pronormoblasts in a bone marrow sample of an AIDS patient with aplastic anemia.

[1 (E) 2 (D) 3 (B) 4 (C. This is seen with erythema infectiosum—also known as Fifth disease.) 5 (F. Ribavirin is active against hepatitis C in combination with interferon alpha.) 6 (D) 7 (E) 8 (A) 9 (C)]

15) A. Acute bacterial endocarditis.
    B. Subacute bacterial endocarditis.
    C. Both.
    D. Neither.

1. Nontender macules on the palms and soles.
2. Pale retinal lesions surrounded by hemorrhage.
3. Tender nodules on the palms, fingertips, and sole.
4. CHF is the most common cause of death.
5. More common on the left side of the heart.
6. 95% of blood cultures are positive.
7. *Staph aureus* is the most common infecting organism.
8. Associated CHF is an indication for surgery.
9. Usually occurs in patients with underlying heart disease.
10. Prosthetic valve endocarditis.

[1 (A; Janeway lesions) 2 (B; Roth spots) 3 (B; Osler nodes) 4 (C) 5 (B) 6 (C) 7 (A) 8 (C) 9 (B) 10 (C)]

16) Brain abscess:
    A. *Nocardia*.
    B. Pneumococcus and *H. influenzae*.
    C. *Taenia solium*.
    D. *Toxoplasma*.

1. Suspect in frontal lobe abscess.
2. Most common cause in immunodeficient patients.
3. Seeds via a pulmonary infection.
4. Child with history of multiple ear infections presents with a brain abscess.
5. Most common cause in developing countries.
6. Suspect in temporal lobe abscess.

[1 (B. These organisms are common in sinus infections. Especially suspect sinus origin in a frontal lobe abscess.) 2 (D; especially seen in AIDS patients. Multiple ring-enhancing lesions.) 3 (A)
4 (B. These organisms are common in ear infections.) 5 (C. This organism causes cysticercosis.) 6 (B. Temporal lobe abscesses are often caused by local extension from an ear infection.)]

17) Diarrhea
    A. *Clostridium difficile*.
    B. *E. coli*.
    C. *Vibrio*.
    D. *Cryptosporidia*.
    E. *Shigella*.
    F. *Entamoeba histolytica*.

1. Liver abscess.
2. Hemolytic-uremic syndrome.
3. Seafood and shellfish.
4. Relapse with this diarrhea is treated with the same antibiotic as used in the initial treatment.
5. < 100 organisms will result in bloody diarrhea.
6. Diagnosed with acid-fast stain of the stool.

[1 (F) 2 (B. This is *E. coli* serotype O157:H7.) 3 (C) 4 (A. This is because it is usually due to the spores becoming active.) 5 (E) 6 (D)]

18) Causes of genital ulceration with regional lymphadenopathy:
    A. Syphilis.
    B. *Granuloma inguinale*.
    C. Herpes Simplex Virus (HSV) infection.
    D. *Lymphogranuloma venereum* (LGV).
    E. Chancroid.

1. Terrible looking painless ulcers.
2. Tender genital nodules that become ulcers. Tender, draining regional lymph nodes.
3. Tender grouped vesicles. Regional lymphadenopathy does not always develop.
4. Single ulcer with raised border. Painless.
5. Single, painless papule/ulcer. Regional lymphadenopathy develops after the ulcer resolves.
6. *Chlamydia trachomatis*.
7. *Klebsiella granulomatis*.
8. *Haemophilus ducreyi*.

[1 (B) 2 (E) 3 (C) 4 (A) 5 (D) 6 (D) 7 (B) 8 (E)]

19) A. Blocks DNA replication.
    B. Blocks supercoiling of DNA.
    C. Blocks transcription of DNA to mRNA.
    D. Reversibly inhibits ribosomal synthesis.
    E. Irreversibly inhibits ribosomal synthesis.

1. Quinolones.
2. Tetracycline, erythromycin, clindamycin, and chloramphenicol.
3. Rifampin.
4. Aminoglycosides.
5. Trimethoprim and sulfonamides.

[1 (B) 2 (D) 3 (C) 4 (E) 5 (A)]

20) General antibacterial properties of the cephalosporins.
    A. 1st generation.
    B. 2nd generation.
    C. 3rd generation.
    D. All of the above.

1. Most resistant to beta lactamase.
2. Active against *Pseudomonas*.
3. Most *Staph*, most *Strep*, not *B. fragilis*.
4. Use with vancomycin for empiric treatment of meningitis
5. Contains the best cephalosporin for anaerobic infections, including those caused by *B. fragilis*.
6. Group of cephalosporins that is most effective against *Staph aureus*.

[1 (C) 2 (C; especially ceftazidime (Fortaz®, Ceptaz®, Tazicef®) 3 (A) 4 (C. Ceftriaxone (Rocephin®), cefotaxime (Claforan®). Remember: In empiric therapy, if the patient is newborn, elderly, or pregnant, ampicillin must be added to cover for *Listeria*.) 5 (B; cefoxitin) 6 (A)]

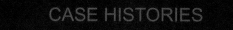

CASE HISTORIES

21) A patient presents with fever, diarrhea, diffuse erythema, and hypocalcemia; what condition do you suspect?

    A Toxic shock syndrome.
    B. Red man syndrome.
    C. Scarlet fever.

[A]

22) If a sheep farmer presents with a history of painless papules, which vesiculated and formed ulcers, and he now has nontender black eschars with nontender induration and swelling, what would you suspect as the cause?

    A. Leptospirosis.
    B. Brucellosis.
    C. Tularemia.
    D. Anthrax.
    E. Plague.

[D]

23) What causative organism is suspected in a camper who presents with constitutional symptoms, flea bites, and lymphadenopathy? Which organism is more likely if this patient is from Arkansas and has tick bites?

    A. Bartonellosis. Plague.
    B. Plague. Tularemia.
    C. Tularemia. Plague.
    D. Plague. Bartonellosis.
    E. Tularemia. Bartonellosis.
    F. Bartonellosis. Tularemia.

[B. Tularemia is similar to plague except plague is transmitted by flea bites and is more common in the desert SW. Bartonellosis is a disease acquired from sandflies in the Andes Mountains. It causes a febrile hemolytic anemia ("Oroya fever").]

24) A feather plucker presents to you with pneumonia and splenomegaly, what do you suspect as being the cause?

    A. Acute candidiasis.
    B. Psittacosis.
    C. Coccidioidomycosis.
    D. Histoplasmosis.
    E. Sporotrichosis.

[B]

25) What do you suspect in the patient who presents with the same symptoms as in the previous question, but with no history of contact with birds? Use the same answers as the previous question.

[D. Although *Histoplasma* is found in bird and bat droppings, most people have no history of contact with birds.]

26) A patient who is a frequent camper presents with fever, arthralgias, and a rash that started in the distal extremities as maculopapular but now is petechial. What is the proper treatment?

    A. Tetracycline.
    B. Penicillin VK.
    C. Third generation cephalosporin.
    D. TMP/SMX.
    E. Clindamycin.
    F. Immune globulin.

[A. This patient has Rocky Mountain spotted fever; this can also be treated with doxycycline or chloramphenicol.]

27) If a hiker presents with foot drop, what infectious disease would you consider?

    A. Syphilis.
    B. *Ehrlichia canis* infection.
    C. Lyme disease.
    D. Rocky Mountain spotted fever.
    E. Plague.
    F. Brucellosis.

[C]

28) A patient presents with a painless chancre on his penis. VDRL is positive. What is the proper treatment?

    A. Benzathine PCN G 2.4 MU IM q week x 3 or doxycycline 100 mg PO bid x 4 weeks
    B. PCN G 12–24 MU IV qd for 10–14 days.
    C. Procaine PCN 2-4 MU IM q d with probenecid 500 mg tid for 14 days
    D. Benzathine PCN G 2.4 MU IM x 1 dose or doxycycline 100 mg bid for 14 days
    E. Doxycycline 100 mg bid x 1 month.

[D. This is also the treatment for the early latency period of secondary syphilis (< 1 year since acquiring the disease). The treatment for late latency of secondary syphilis is given in A. The answers given in B and C are means of treating neurosyphilis; doxycycline is an alternative for the non-pregnant penicillin-allergic patient; for pregnancy, desensitization is the correct answer.]

29) A patient presents with a severe cellulitis of the face. Blood cultures are done, and the patient is placed on oral cloxacillin. 2 days later the infection appears to be worse and he has fever to 102° F. Preliminary results of the blood culture show a coagulase-negative *Staph*. What should be done next?

  A. Nothing; it often takes 2–3 days to notice any change with severe cellulitis.
  B. Repeat blood cultures and change the antibiotic to IV erythromycin.
  C. Repeat blood cultures and change to IV ceftriaxone.
  D. Repeat blood cultures and change to IV cefazolin.
  E. Change the antibiotic to oral ciprofloxacin.
  F. Change the antibiotic to oral TMP/SMX.

[D. Trick question. *S. epidermidis* infections never present this way (think more infected indwelling catheter). The likelihood that the blood culture represents a contaminant is > 90%. In the era of community-acquired MRSA, this organism also must be considered, but IV vancomycin was not given as a choice, so the best choice is to begin parenteral therapy against the most likely organisms, *Staphylococcus aureus* and *Streptococcus pyogenes*.]

30) An AIDS patient presents with signs and symptoms of meningitis. Which of the following organisms is both a likely cause in this patient and is highly unlikely to occur in an immunocompetent patient?

  A. *Bacillus cereus*.
  B. *S. aureus*.
  C. *Listeria monocytogenes*.
  D. *Cryptococcus neoformans*.
  E. *Corynebacterium jeikeium*.
  F. *S. agalactiae*.

[D]

31) If a diabetic patient of yours presents with a black, necrotic spot in the nose and complaining of headache, what disease entity would you suspect?

  A. Ecthyma gangrenosum.
  B. Anthrax.
  C. Rhinocerebral mucormycosis.

[C. Rhinocerebral mucormycosis has a very poor prognosis. Ecthyma gangrenosum (round indurated black lesion with central ulceration) is seen with pseudomonal bacteremia. The cutaneous form of anthrax starts as a painless papule that vesiculates and forms a painless ulcer and then a painless black eschar, often with a lot of nonpitting, painless induration and swelling.]

32) A patient presents 1 month after an eco-tour of the Amazon rain forests. He is complaining of shaking chills and fever. His family tells you he has episodes of hallucination. His urine shows nephrotic-range proteinuria. What is the treatment for this patient?

  A. Sodium stibogluconate.
  B. Pyrimethamine and sulfadiazine.
  C. Clindamycin.
  D. Chloroquine and primaquine.
  E. Chloroquine alone.
  F. Metronidazole

[E. All the types of malaria can cause nephritis from immune complex deposition. *P. malariae* is the one most commonly associated with nephrotic syndrome. It is usually treated with chloroquine only. *P. vivax* and *P. ovale* require the additional primaquine. Sodium stibogluconate is used to treat leishmaniasis. Metronidazole: *Giardia*, *Trichomonas*, and amebiasis. Pyrimethamine and sulfadiazine: toxoplasmosis. Clindamycin: babesiosis.]

33) If a patient from south Texas presents with a large liver abscess, which, when aspirated, shows no amoeba or PMNs, how would it be treated?

  A. Sodium stibogluconate.
  B. Pyrimethamine and sulfadiazine.
  C. Quinacrine.
  D. Clindamycin.
  E. Chloroquine and primaquine.
  F. Chloroquine alone.
  G. Metronidazole.

[G. This patient has amebiasis. The *Entamoeba histolytica* is usually not seen in the liver abscess aspirate.]

34) A patient being treated with ganciclovir for a severe CMV infection develops neutropenia and thrombocytopenia. What is a possible cause?

  A. Ganciclovir.
  B. The CMV infection itself.
  C. The combination of the infection and ganciclovir.
  D. All of the above.
  E. It is related to neither the infection nor ganciclovir.

[D. The major toxicity of ganciclovir is bone marrow toxicity (30%!!) resulting in neutropenia and thrombocytopenia. CMV infection itself can cause bone marrow suppression as well.]

35) If a woman who has been pregnant 2 months presents with a measles-looking rash and the hemagglutination inhibition test is negative, what is the next step that should be done?

  A. Start ribavirin therapy.
  B. Check for inclusion bodies in the skin scraping.
  C. Repeat the test again in 3 weeks.
  D. Give the measles vaccine.
  E. Therapeutic abortion.

[C. The hemagglutination inhibition test is used to diagnose Rubella (German measles). If it is negative in a newly exposed pregnant patient, repeat the test again in 3 weeks (i.e., after the incubation period). If it is then positive, therapeutic abortion should be considered. Ribavirin is used in combination with interferon alpha for hepatitis C. Inclusion bodies found in a BAL specimen are pathognomonic for CMV pneumonitis.]

37) A sickle cell patient presents with extreme fatigue and weakness. Diagnosis is aplastic anemia. The bone marrow biopsy also shows giant pronormoblast cells. What is the probable etiology?

   A. Parvovirus infection.
   B. Sickle cell burnout after a nonspecific viral infection.
   C. Acute myelogenous leukemia.
   D. Retrovirus infection.
   E. Norovirus (Norwalk virus) infection.
   F. Rhinovirus infection.

[A. Parvovirus infection can cause aplastic anemia in patients with hemolytic anemia or with AIDS. Norovirus (Norwalk virus): winter vomiting disease. Retroviruses: HTLV-1 = T-cell leukemia; HTLV-2 = a T-cell variant of hairy cell leukemia; HIV = AIDS. Rhinoviruses: main cause of URIs.]

38) A patient presents with a thin "skim milk" vaginal discharge, clue cells, and a positive whiff test. What is the diagnosis?

   A. Bacterial vaginosis.
   B. Yeast vaginitis.
   C. *Chlamydia* infection.
   D. Gonorrhea.
   E. *Trichomonas vaginalis* vaginitis.

[A. Bacterial vaginosis is treated with a 7-day course of metronidazole or clindamycin.]

39) A patient presents with a frothy vaginal discharge, no clue cells, a positive whiff test, and a strawberry cervix. What is the diagnosis?

   A. Bacterial vaginosis.
   B. Yeast vaginitis.
   C. *Chlamydia* infection.
   D. Gonorrhea.
   E. *Trichomonas vaginalis* vaginitis.

[E. *Trichomonas vaginalis* vaginitis is treated with 1 dose of metronidazole. Notice that both this type of vaginitis and bacterial vaginosis have a positive whiff test, but only bacterial vaginosis has the clue cells. Note: buzz phrase for trichomoniasis is "strawberry cervix."]

40) A patient presents with a mucoid cervical discharge. Gram stain of the discharge shows only WBCs. What is the treatment?

   A. Procaine penicillin 2.4 million units IM.
   B. Benzathine penicillin 2.4 million units IM.
   C. Doxycycline 100 mg PO bid for 10 days.
   D. Metronidazole 500 mg PO tid for 7 days.
   E. Ceftriaxone 1 gram IM.

[C. The most likely cause of this is *Chlamydia*. Gonorrhea has not been ruled out, but of the choices given, C is the best.]

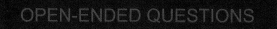
OPEN-ENDED QUESTIONS

41) What are the 3 different types of growth factors? How do these substances work?

[Growth factor is the newer name for the substances, which include interleukins, colony-stimulating factors, and erythropoietin. These substances are the actual molecules, which stimulate the cells by combining with the cell surface receptors.]

42) Another class of cytokines, the interferons, have 3 types: alpha, beta, and gamma. Which one is the most potent and what cell type produces it?

[The most potent interferon in the immune system is gamma, which is produced by T cells (both helper and suppressor).]

43) In neutropenic patients on bone marrow transplant wards, *Corynebacterium jeikeium* is an important cause of infections. What is the most common cause of infection in neutropenic patients? What are some of the other causes of infection in these patients?

[Infections in neutropenic patients are usually due to Gram-negative bacilli, but *Staphylococcus aureus* is also common, and infections due to *S. epidermidis* and fungi (*Candida*, *Aspergillus*, and *Mucor*) also may occur.]

44) Beta-lactam antibiotics are not generally used as the sole antibiotic for neutropenic patients with documented infection. Why?

[Rapid development of resistance to beta-lactams by Gram-negative organisms.]

45) How is it that AIDS patients also have a humoral deficiency?

[The decrease in CD4 cells decreases the normal suppressive effect that CD4 cells have on B cells, and there is an overproduction of nonspecific immunoglobulins—which "gum up the works."]

46) A loss of what organ increases the severity of babesiosis?

[The spleen.]

47) In an atopic patient with frequent bouts of otitis media and giardiasis, what humoral deficiency do you suspect?

[IgA deficiency.]

48) What type of immune deficiency do you suspect in someone with frequent bouts of low-grade meningococcemia?

[Late complement deficiency.]

49) In what diseases are patients T-cell–deficient?

[AIDS, Hodgkin lymphoma, and T-cell ALL. Also patients on steroids or alkylating agents or post-transplant.]

50) What previous infections might reactivate in a person with impaired cellular immunity?

[*Nocardia*, TB, *Cryptococcus*, blastomycosis, histoplasmosis, coccidioidomycosis, and *Strongyloides*.]

51) Name 4 factors that account for, or increase, the pathogenicity of the staphylococcus bacteria.

[Enterotoxin, exotoxin, coagulase, and leukocidin.]

52) What type of *S. pneumoniae* is usually the most virulent and with what protein is this virulence associated?

[Type 3; M protein.]

53) In what patient groups are you most likely to find an infection caused by *Strep agalactiae*?

[The neonates and the elderly (especially if alcoholic or diabetic).]

54) In what patient groups do infections caused by *Listeria monocytogenes* occur?

[The elderly, neonates, and pregnant women.]

55) What type of infection is most likely after a TURP? How do you treat it?

[*Enterococcus*. Treat with ampicillin or penicillin plus gentamicin or if resistant to penicillin use vancomycin; if it is VRE, use tigecycline or quinupristin/dalfopristin.]

56) In what way is the treatment for *Listeria monocytogenes* infection similar to that for enterococcal infections?

[Both *Listeria* and enterococci are resistant to all cephalosporins. Both are treated with an aminoglycoside and penicillin or ampicillin.]

57) If a patient presents with hoarseness, sore throat, and a low-grade fever, what would you suspect as the cause? What if he also had a gray-white pharyngeal membrane? What is the treatment of choice for this organism?

[Viral syndrome. Diphtheria. Erythromycin.]

58) In what situation is *Corynebacterium jeikeium* especially a problem?

[On bone marrow transplant units.]

59) If a patient comes in with sepsis caused by *Clostridium septicum*, what other workup is required?

[GI malignancy workup; usually a colonoscopy is the choice.]

60) What is the main toxin in all *Clostridia*?

[Alpha toxin.]

61) Name 2 immune deficiencies in which infection by *Neisseria meningitidis* is more common.

[Humoral deficiencies and late complement deficiencies. Also those without functioning spleens are at increased risk.]

62) Where does *Salmonella typhi* tend to seed in chronic carriers?

[In the gallbladder.]

63) In what patient group do you expect to see *Moraxella catarrhalis* respiratory infections?

[In patients with COPD and those with immunodeficiencies.]

64) What are buboes?

[Very large lymph nodes (as in bubonic plague).]

65) What type of *Chlamydia* is associated with neonatal eye infections and neonatal pneumonia?

[*C. trachomatis*.]

66) In which type of septic shock does the patient have warm extremities?

[Gram-negative.]

67) How long after primary syphilis does secondary syphilis occur? What percentage of untreated secondary syphilis goes on to tertiary syphilis?

[~ 2 months. ~ 33%]

68) Of the 2 general types of serologic tests for syphilis, the non-treponemal and the specific treponemal, which type is positive in a neonate whose mother was positive?

[Both the specific treponemal and non-treponemal tests are positive; they are IgG antibodies, which can pass across the placenta.]

69) What organism is especially associated with septic peripheral thrombophlebitis and septic thrombosis of the great central veins?

[*Candida albicans*.]

70) Is amphotericin B a good choice for ringworm?

[No.]

71) Of the 2 main types of parasites (protozoa and helminths), which causes eosinophilia? Which are single-celled? Which tend to replicate within the body?

[Helminths. Protozoa. Protozoa.]

72) How is the diagnosis of acute toxoplasmosis made?

[Elevated specific IgM antibody or in an AIDS patient by finding "ring enhancing" lesions on an MRI of the brain.]

73) Which RBC antigen is the site of attachment for *P. vivax*?

[The Duffy RBC antigen.]

74) What does the protozoan *Babesia microti* have in common with *Borrelia burgdorferi*? What does it have in common with malaria?

[Both *Babesia microti* and *Borrelia burgdorferi* are transmitted by the *Ixodes* tick. Both *Babesia microti* and the *Plasmodia* are intra-RBC parasites.]

75) What is the only helminth that replicates in the body?

[*Strongyloides* is the only common helminth that replicates in the body.]

76) What is the drug of choice for any type of *Schistosoma* infection?

[Praziquantel.]

77) Which lab result is pathognomonic for herpes zoster infection?

[Multinucleated giant cells in a skin scraping.]

78) Does prednisone given in the treatment for herpes zoster help decrease the incidence of post-herpetic neuralgia?

[No, randomized trials have confirmed that the addition of prednisone to anti-HSV therapy does not decrease the incidence or the duration of post-herpetic neuralgia. However, prednisone has been shown to improve ACUTE neuralgia and diminish need for analgesics, especially in those > 50 years of age.]

79) What type of cells are the atypical lymphs found in a patient with infectious mononucleosis?

[T cells.]

80) How is Epstein-Barr (EB) virus associated with the hairy leukoplakia seen in early HIV disease?

[EB virus causes hairy leukoplakia.]

81) Which virus is ribavirin effective against?

[Ribavirin is treatment of choice for hepatitis C in combination with interferon alpha. It has some activity against influenza A & B, but flu vaccine, oseltamivir (Tamiflu®—oral) and zanamivir (Relenza®—powder for inhalation) are preferred treatments or prophylactic agents.]

82) What type of virus are oral amantadine and rimantadine effective against?

[None. The correct answer used to be influenza A, but beginning with the 2005-2006 influenza season, influenza A became widely resistant to both of these agents.]

83) In a nursing home threatened by influenza A, what should be done?

[The patients, staff, and physicians should all be immunized and then take oseltamivir for 2 weeks (until adequate antibodies have formed from immunization).]

84) What variants of papillomavirus are associated with cervical cancer?

[16, 18, and 31.]

85) What virus causes progressive multifocal leukoencephalopathy? In what patient group is this usually seen?

[Papovavirus is reactivated in AIDS patients and causes progressive multifocal leukoencephalopathy in this group.]

86) How do you differentiate mumps from bacterial parotitis?

[Gram stain the parotid secretions. Bacterial parotitis has many WBCs in the secretions, whereas mumps has none.]

87) What are the CD4-positive cells in which HIV replicates?

[Helper T cells, monocytes, and macrophages.]

88) What causes the polyclonal increase in serum immune-globulins in AIDS patients?

[The CD4+ helper T cells decrease and no longer tonically suppress the B lymphocytes.]

89) When is antibody to HIV detectable after the initial inoculation? How is this antibody detected?

[Within 1–3 months after the initial inoculation, the anti-HIV antibody is detectable by the ELISA test.]

90) What is the significance of the P24 HIV antigen?

[This is an HIV core protein that is an early detectable sign of HIV infection; it is no longer clinically useful and has been supplanted by HIV PCR DNA and RNA testing.]

91) What is the most common lung disease in AIDS patients?

[Pneumocystis Pneumonia (PCP).]

92) At what CD4 count is prophylaxis for PCP started?

[< 200.]

93) Which of the drugs used to treat PCP causes neutropenia? Which causes skin rash? Which causes hypoglycemia?

[Neutropenia: TMP/SMX (Bactrim) and pentamidine. Skin rash: TMP/SMX. Hyperglycemia or hypoglycemia: pentamidine.]

94) Why is pyrimethamine + sulfadoxine (Fansidar®) not used much in prophylaxis for PCP?

[Because it (rarely) causes Stevens-Johnson syndrome and is much more expensive than TMP/SMX.]

95) Histoplasmosis or coccidioidomycosis: Which one causes arthralgias? Which one causes splenomegaly?

[Arthralgias: coccidioidomycosis. Splenomegaly: histoplasmosis.]

96) What are two side effects of ddI therapy in an AIDS patient?

[Pancreatitis and peripheral neuropathy are the most commonly tested on.]

97) If a patient with AIDS, Hodgkin disease, or diabetes develops meningitis, what test must be done on the CSF in addition to the usual CSF survey?

[Cryptococcal antigen (or India ink).]

98) If the blood cultures are negative in bacterial endocarditis, what organisms are the most likely cause?

[Previoulsy it was thought one of the HACEK organisms would be likely: *Haemophilus, Actinobacillus, Cardiobacterium, Eikenella*, and *Kingella*. However in the modern microbiologic era, fastidious organisms (zoonotic agents and fungi) and streptococcal species, especially in those who have received previous antibiotic therapy are the most common causes of culture-negative endocarditis, a prospective study showed *Coxiella burnetii* was found in 48%, *Bartonella* in 28%]

99) When is surgery required in bacterial endocarditis?

[When there is fistula, abscess, pericarditis, or persistent fever, and in cases when the resulting valve dysfunction causes heart failure. Also, when there is a conduction disturbance in a patient with aortic valve endocarditis.]

100) What is the most common cause of death due to endocarditis?

[Ventricular failure.]

101) Name the organisms that most commonly cause acute native valve bacterial endocarditis.

[*Staph aureus* (40%), pneumococci, Group A *Strep*, enterococci, and then Gram-negative organisms and *S. epidermidis*.]

102) What is the only common peripheral manifestation of ABE?

[Janeway spots (nontender macules on the palms and soles).]

103) What are the peripheral manifestations of subacute bacterial endocarditis (SBE)?

[Roth spots (pale retinal lesions surrounded by hemorrhage), petechiae, splinter hemorrhages, and Osler nodes (small tender nodules on the palms, fingertips, and soles).]

104) If a patient presents 45 days after a prosthetic valve insertion and has signs and symptoms of endocarditis, what would be the most likely next step: surgery or intensive medical therapy?

[Early prosthetic valve endocarditis (< 60 days) is usually due to seeding during surgery. It has an acute presentation and requires emergent surgery.]

105) What organism that causes prosthetic valve endocarditis can sometimes be cured by antibiotics alone?

[Viridans Streptococci endocarditis. This usually presents subacutely and > 60 days after surgery.]

106) What organisms do you suspect in a chronic meningitis with a neutrophilic CSF?

[*Nocardia, Actinomyces,* or fungus.]

107) What is the most common cause of acute encephalitis?

[Unknown! Although it is thought to be viral.]

108) What is the procedure of choice for diagnosing brain abscesses? What is the most common cause of brain abscess in developing countries? What is the empiric therapy for presumed bacterial brain abscesses?

[CT scan. Cysticercosis (from ingesting eggs of the pork tapeworm, *Taenia solium*) is the most common cause in developing countries. Usually a 3rd generation cephalosporin (cefotaxime or ceftriaxone) plus metronidazole. If MRSA is suspected or is a post-neurological procedure, then add vancomycin.]

109) What is the test of choice for diagnosing neurosyphilis? Why is a CSF FTA-ABS not used to diagnose neurosyphilis?

[CSF-VDRL (100% specific, 50% sensitive). The CSF FTA-ABS is so sensitive that a positive result can be due to contamination of the sample by peripheral blood.]

110) 5% of healthy persons have *C. difficile* in their stool. How can you tell if the diarrhea is caused by *C. difficile*?

[A *C. difficile* cytotoxin assay is done, not a culture.]

111) What viruses cause severe diarrhea in infants?

[Rotavirus is the most common cause of severe diarrhea in infants.]

112) What viruses are associated with diarrhea after eating clams or oysters and also associated with cruise ship outbreaks?

[Norovirus (Norwalk virus). This is called "winter vomiting disease." The Noroviruses are identified by the stool ELISA test.]

113) Why is a brush often used in obtaining a cervical *Chlamydia* culture?

[Because *Chlamydia* are intracellular parasites, and cells from the cervix are required for diagnosis.]

114) How is gonococcal urethritis diagnosed?

[Positive culture or an exudate Gram-stain showing Gram-negative, intra-WBC diplococci.]

115) What are the causative organisms in non-GC urethritis?

[*Chlamydia trachomatis*, *Ureaplasma urealyticum*, *Trichomonas vaginalis*, and HSV.]

116) What is the treatment for non-GC urethritis?

[Azithromycin or doxycycline. Erythromycin if pregnant.]

117) What does the skin rash of disseminated gonococcemia look like?

[It usually consists of a few lesions that are papular with hemorrhage into the papules (very red papules).]

118) What is the best way of making the diagnosis of disseminated gonococcemia?

[Gram stain and C&S of the lesions and all body orifices results in an 85% yield.]

119) How is menstruation associated with severity of symptoms in a GC infection with gonococcemia?

[Severity of symptoms is increased.]

120) What is the pH of the vaginal fluid in the following situations: normal, yeast vaginitis, trichomoniasis, bacterial vaginosis.

[Normal and yeast vaginitis: < 4.5. Trichomoniasis and bacterial vaginosis: > 5.0.]

121) What are the risk factors in women for UTI?

[Sexual activity, spermicide-diaphragm use, and insulin-treated diabetes.]

122) What is the indication to treat a woman with symptoms of acute cystitis and no complicating factors?

[Pyuria alone is an indication to treat in this patient group.]

123) Should asymptomatic bacteriuria be treated in pregnant women? What if it occurs in neutropenic patients? Transplant patients? If there is an indwelling Foley catheter? In a nursing home patient?

[Asymptomatic bacteriuria (> 10^5) should be treated in pregnant patients (1/3 go on to pyelonephritis!), neutropenic patients, diabetics, and transplant patients. It is not treated in elderly patients or patients with Foley catheters. However, in elderly patients with symptomatic bacteriuria you always treat!]

124) Why should TMP/SMX (Bactrim®, Septra®, Sulfatrim®) not be given in late pregnancy?

[TMP/SMX is not given in late pregnancy or early nursing mothers because it can cause kernicterus in the child.]

125) Why do the lesions caused by *Mycobacterium marinum* often localize in the distal extremities?

[Because the organism does not grow well at body temperature.]

126) If an IV drug abuser presents with osteomyelitis of the spine, what is the probable causative organism?

[Think *Pseudomonas* in this patient group, especially if the infection involves the spine or pelvis. MRSA would also be on the differential.]

127) Does a negative pyrophosphate scan exclude osteomyelitis?

[Yes, a negative pyrophosphate scan excludes osteomyelitis. A positive scan can be caused by other infections and with bone fractures.]

128) What is the order of frequency of nosocomial infections?

[UTI > post-op wound infections > pneumonia.]

129) What is the most common organism to cause a UTI in a 60-year-old woman?

[*E. coli.*]

130) What is the most common vector of nosocomial disease between patients in the ICU?

[Hands of the ICU workers.]

131) What are the common and uncommon causes of IV catheter-related infections?

[Common: *S. aureus* and *S. epidermidis*. Less common: *Candida*, *Corynebacterium jeikeium* and *Bacillus cereus*.]

132) Why is nafcillin used in lieu of methicillin?

[Methicillin is associated with interstitial nephritis.]

133) Why, even though penicillin is the drug of choice for meningococcal infections, is rifampin or ciprofloxacin used for eradication of the carrier state?

[Because they concentrate in the upper respiratory mucosa.]

134) Which is the 2nd generation cephalosporin that is useful in treating meningitis?

None. Only 3rd and 4th generations are now approved for treatment of meningitis.

135) Which of the cephalosporins are active against *Pseudomonas*?

[The 3rd generation cephalosporin, ceftazidime (Fortaz$^{®}$) and the 4th generation cefepime (Maxipime$^{®}$]

136) Which of the 3rd generation cephalosporins cross an inflamed blood-brain barrier?

[Ceftriaxone, cefotaxime, and ceftazidime. Note: Only ceftriaxone and cefotaxime are used with vancomycin for empiric treatment of meningitis pending results of CSF analysis (if patients are neonates, elderly, or pregnant, ampicillin is added to also cover for *Listeria*). Ceftazidime does not have enough Gram-positive coverage anymore to be reliable for any strain of *S. pneumoniae*.]

137) Why is ciprofloxacin not recommended for the routine treatment of community-acquired pneumonia?

[Because today there is marked *S. pneumoniae* resistance]

138) Name some of the broadest-spectrum antibiotics and what are their spectrum?

[Imipenem, meropenem, doripenem, and cefepime. They are effective against most bacteria. The organisms resistant to them can include *Enterococcus faecium*, *Pseudomonas cepacia*, *Corynebacterium jeikeium*, *Xanthomonas maltophilia*, and methicillin-resistant *Staphylococci*.]

139) Explain the mechanisms of the beta-lactamase inhibitors: sulbactam and clavulanic acid.

[These inhibitors bind irreversibly to the beta-lactamase made by the bacteria.]

140) What is "red man syndrome"?

[Red man syndrome is a **non-allergic** reaction to vancomycin, which causes tachycardia, flushing, pruritus, and sometimes angioedema. It results from the release of histamine from mast cells usually because of a too rapid infusion of vancomycin.]

141) Which antibiotics have a persistent anti-Gram–negative effect after removal of the drug (also known as the post-antibiotic effect)?

[Aminoglycosides and fluoroquinolones.]

142) Which cephalosporin is effective against *Listeria*?

[None. Penicillin or ampicillin is the drug of choice.]

143) Why is azithromycin a drug of choice for community-acquired pneumonias?

[Because azithromycin is effective against *Mycoplasma pneumoniae*, *S. pneumoniae*, and *Chlamydophila pneumoniae*.]

144) Why is rifampin never given alone to treat an acute infection?

[Because organisms rapidly develop resistance to rifampin.]

145) What is the main toxicity of ganciclovir?

[Bone marrow toxicity.]

NOTES

NOTES